CARING *for* YOUR CHILD *with* SEVERE FOOD ALLERGIES

*Emotional Support and
Practical Advice from
a Parent Who's Been There*

∾

Lisa Cipriano Collins,
M.A., M.F.T.

John Wiley & Sons, Inc.
New York • Chichester • Weinheim • Brisbane • Singapore • Toronto

This book is printed on acid-free paper. ∞

Copyright © 2000 by Lisa Cipriano Collins. All rights reserved

Published by John Wiley & Sons, Inc.
Published simultaneously in Canada

Illustrations on pages 41 and 43 courtesy of Victoria Schubert, Press1

Design and production by Navta Associates, Inc.

The information contained in this book is not intended to serve as a replacement for professional medical advice. Any use of the information in this book is at the reader's discretion. The author and the publisher specifically disclaim any and all liability arising directly or indirectly from the use or application of any information contained in this book. A health care professional should be consulted regarding your specific situation.

Library of Congress Cataloging-in-Publication Data:

Collins, Lisa Cipriano.
    Caring for your child with severe food allergies : emotional support and practical advice from a parent who's been there / Lisa Cipriano Collins.
        p.   cm.
    Includes bibliographical references and index.
    ISBN 0-471-34785-X
    1. Food allergy in children Popular works.   I. Title.
RJ386.5.C64   1999
618.92'975—dc21   99-15192

Printed in the United States of America

10 9 8 7 6 5 4 3 2 1

CARING *for* YOUR CHILD *with* SEVERE FOOD ALLERGIES

I DEDICATE THIS BOOK TO MY FAMILY. To my husband, Billy, for always having more love for me and more faith in my potential than even I dared to dream. To my son, Max: Without you I never would have seen the need to write this book. You have taught me so much. I'm so proud to watch you grow and mature; you are so confident and thoughtful in how you manage every aspect of your life. To my daughter Emily: Your spark of independence has surprised me since the day you were born. Now your independence mixes so beautifully with your immense capacity for love and caring. It inspires me, and you have taught me all over again how to be female. And last but not least to my baby daughter, Ruby: Your sweetness has brought a deep joy into my life that I never knew was possible. I love you all.

~

CONTENTS

———— ～ ————

ACKNOWLEDGMENTS

———— 〜 ————

I AM GRATEFUL to my fellow students, my teachers, and my supervisors who, over the course of my education, have contributed to my personal growth and have made me feel empowered to write this important book. I wish to acknowledge in particular the help and support of Daphne Davidson, Charlotte Rodgers, Jane Burgess, Maryjo Barnett, and the staff of the Burlington Community Life Center.

I also wish to recognize people who have made it possible for me to take the time and energy necessary to complete this work. I thank my husband, Billy, for his never-ending patience and support. The active role he takes in parenting our three children has been vital to my success. And I thank my mom, Josephine Cipriano, who has always been there for me in every way.

I would also like to thank all the people who helped out with my children on days when I desperately needed to continue my work. They include Joan Frederick, Shelly Pariseau, Annmarie Roche, Cathy O'Neil, Nicole Gagnon, and Denise and Ricki Lane. I would also like to acknowledge all my son's teachers and his school nurse, who have opened their hearts and minds to us in keeping Max safe at school. His school nurse, Joanne Ferrick, gave me the peace of mind that enabled me to try to help others in the same predicament. Thanks also to my son's pediatrician, Lawrence Hoder, M.D., and his allergist, John Saryan, M.D., who provide the best possible health care.

For their ability to simultaneously challenge and support me, I wish to thank Marion Nesbit, Debbie Slobodnik, and Linda Perruzzi. They played a key role in unlocking my potential. I would also like to thank Anne Russell, Rosemarie Tieri, Ellie Goldberg, Helen Penney, Gloria Collins, Susan Collins, Victoria Schubert, and Maggie Plasse for the important role they each played at various points in this project.

I would like to thank those involved in the publishing process, starting with Michael Valentino, my literary agent from Cambridge Literary Associates. He kindly agreed to take on this first-time author as a client and enthusiastically succeeded in finding this book a publisher. Thanks to Cheryl Kimball, who recognized that this was a book worth pursuing, to Jeff Braun who did an amazing editing job, and finally to Betsy Thorpe and Sibylle Kazeroid of John Wiley & Sons for the ongoing expert care they have provided to me and my manuscript in the final stages of the editing and production process.

I would also like to formally acknowledge Anne Muñoz-Furlong, the founder and president of the Food Allergy Network, who generously shared much of the information contained here. Her dedication and personal sacrifice cannot be understated, as her network continues to help its members, numbering in the tens of thousands, in so many ways. Last, and by no means least important, I would like to thank the parents of food-allergic children who participated in a lengthy informal survey as well as follow-up interviews. My questions were not easy to face. My hope is that by sharing our stories here, we will be helping many, many families who follow in our footsteps.

INTRODUCTION

───────── ∼ ─────────

IN THE UNITED STATES, an estimated 6 percent of children—4 million children—are affected by true food allergies, according to the Food Allergy Network, with a higher prevalence in boys than girls. I emphasize *true* food allergies because reactions to food are not always due to an allergy. (More on this in chapter 1.) Allergic reactions to food range from hives to nausea and vomiting to anaphylactic shock. *Anaphylaxis* is the term used for the most serious of allergic reactions, which involves one or more body systems. The most serious symptom that may be experienced in anaphylaxis is a rapid and severe drop in blood pressure leading to unconsciousness. Left untreated or undertreated, anaphylaxis can result in death.

When your child runs the risk of dying if he or she eats the wrong food—or is even exposed to it—a normal childhood seems out of the question. Yet balancing safety with normalcy is paramount.

Managing the care of a child at risk for experiencing a food-induced anaphylactic reaction is a family affair. As you know or will discover, parents, siblings, and even caregivers of food-allergic children often carry an emotional burden. Stress can affect family dynamics and threaten the emotional and physical health of everyone, including the food-allergic child.

This book is based on my studies of family systems, as well as our family's experiences and those of other families dealing with

1

food allergies. It is written both for the immediate family of a child with severe food allergies and for extended family members and other caregivers who want to offer the family support. My goal in writing this guide is to help family members minimize the risk to the food-allergic child of experiencing a food-induced anaphylactic reaction, have healthier emotional lives, and be better able to communicate the food-allergic child's needs to others who care for the child in the parents' absence. This guide is also intended to help caregivers become confident about their ability to provide safe care for the food-allergic child and to be better able to communicate with the child's family. They, too, will be able to promote a healthier emotional life for the food-allergic child.

Some of the issues addressed in this book may be of great concern to you at this particular time, while others may not. Some issues may be ongoing. Families say the process of managing a child at risk for anaphylaxis does not present itself as a straight line with a beginning and an end that simply needs to be worked through. Instead, the process seems to have no end. Frequently, issues are revisited as the food-allergic child's environment or stage of development changes. With this in mind, it is my intention through this work to provide a forum for you to visit and revisit the issues that are of particular concern to you and the family.

Please keep in mind that the information contained in this guide is not intended to be a substitute for consultation with the child's physician. All matters of health require medical supervision. Basic food allergy information is presented to empower you to better communicate the child's needs to others, as well as to help you make decisions about practical daily living. This is not a book on the medical management of food allergies.

My hope is that families and caregivers will learn ways to support one another and create an environment in which trust, faith, hope, normalcy, and self-esteem can grow and flourish. Most important, they will learn to increase the level of safety for children with severe food allergies—in and out of their presence.

1

FIRST ENCOUNTERS
WITH A SEVERE FOOD
ALLERGY

———— ∽ ————

IN THE PROCESS of researching this book, I had the privilege of hearing many families' personal food allergy stories. The most profound story almost always seemed to be the answer to that loaded question: "How did you find out about your child's allergy?" I noticed that whenever there were two or more sets of parents of food-allergic children in a room you could count the seconds until one would ask the other this same question. And it is also the question I am most often asked by members of the media and every other person who is aware of my son's allergy.

People's answers seemed to fall into two categories. One group of parents experienced a single event—such as an unexpected and obvious allergic reaction that landed their child in an emergency room—followed by a swift diagnosis. The other group of parents told me of a slower process: of an infant or toddler who experienced many health problems such as colic, gastrointestinal problems, or eczema-like symptoms for a long period of time. After countless doctor appointments or changes in diet and formulas, a diagnosis of true food allergies was finally made.

In either case, the realization that a serious health concern exists for their child is one of the worst things that can happen to parents. Many times parents don't allow themselves to process this trauma because uninformed doctors or family members tell them that all they have to do is avoid the food that their child is allergic to. Well, it sounds simple. Even you may rob yourself of owning what you feel by looking at your otherwise healthy child and telling yourself that it could be so much worse. After all, we are not talking about diabetes or, God forbid, leukemia or some other cancer.

As a parent, you tell yourself that you can handle this, but you soon find that you do not even know where to start. There is no magic formula for managing the safety of your child; after all, he or she must eat! But what is safe? Well-intentioned people may share every horror story they have ever heard of a child, teenager, or adult dying within minutes of eating the food to which they were allergic. My son is allergic to peanuts, and I have heard stories of peanuts being found in chili, in a plain cookie that was cross-contaminated in someone's kitchen, and on the label of all kinds of unlikely items, even *plain* M&M's.

Upon joining the Food Allergy Network, you will start receiving a helpful and indispensable bimonthly newsletter called *Food Allergy News*, as well as special mailings called Alerts, which are sent out each time there is a specific mislabeling or cross-contamination problem. For example, there could be peanuts in the cracker-and-cheese sandwich cookies you bought last week or in your child's favorite cereal. Worse yet, you wonder if the food you are feeding your child today will be the subject of tomorrow's emergency Alert. Then you start thinking about the birthday party your child is invited to and wondering about the safety of your child's environment at day care, school, your neighbor's, or Grandma's house. You realize that you will need to tell all these people about your child's food allergy. You realize that all of these people will need to know how to recognize a reaction and administer an auto-injector of epinephrine. You talk to a friend, sister, teacher, or mother and you quickly realize that many people are not aware of the seriousness of food allergies, and some may even sound as if they do not believe you. In the worst-case scenario, perhaps even your spouse does not share your level of concern.

Perhaps you would not categorize your reaction to your child's diagnosis as being this dramatic. Or perhaps this description does not even begin to address the grief and panic you have felt or are feeling now. Either way, it is my belief from my own experience and the observation of other parents' experiences that it is essential to allow yourself to recognize and feel the effects of the many ways that this diagnosis has affected your and your family's life.

For instance, suddenly there is another consideration to factor into almost every conceivable decision, such as whether my son should be allowed to go to certain birthday parties, play at a new friend's house, or ride to school on the chaotic bus that I imagine is filled to the brim with bullies toting killer peanut butter and jelly sandwiches. Having to do this kind of thinking for every seemingly normal activity can be hard to accept as well as exhausting. My desire to provide my son with a normal life made me want to go on with living and disregard this new consideration so as not to let the allergy "win." What I've found is that living can go on and my son can participate in almost every "normal" activity.

However, in our case, the decision-making process must be different. Simple decisions often become major issues. At first, it simply takes more time and effort to apply this new decision-making process, which can make life feel arduous. You must ask yourself, "Will my child be safe if he participates in this activity?" By the word *activity* I mean anything and everything, from continuing with day care to going out for an ice cream cone or going on an educational overnight with the school. Then you must go on to consider all the variables. Will your child be with someone who knows about the allergy and knows how to recognize and treat a reaction? Will there be food there? Will your child be close to an emergency room, should the need arise? Is your child old enough to handle the inherent risks involved? How much does your child really want to do this? How will your other children feel if you need to accompany your food-allergic child? Can you feel comfortable with the amount of risk involved?

Some of the questions you ask yourself may be hard to answer. It is up to you to consider all the variables and make a decision. Many times you will decide to allow the activity even though it will mean extra work on your part for you to feel confident about the safety of your child. This may mean going out of your way to become a part of the activity yourself, or taking the time to educate another adult who may or may not be willing to help. This sounds like a lot for most parents who may already have a lot going on with family and community life, as well as perhaps working outside the home.

Having to adopt a new way of making decisions can sometimes be overwhelming. Having to live with the honesty of the answers that you arrive at may also be difficult. What if, after honestly evaluating an opportunity, you find that you cannot allow your child to participate in something that you enjoyed as a child? For instance, perhaps you decide that the risk of cross-contamination at ice cream parlors is too high and you will no longer stop at your family's favorite ice cream shop on the way home from the beach. How will you experience that loss? How will you deal with the possible anger from your child? How will this decision affect your other children, and how will you deal with their feelings? Some parents tend to respond to their new reality by feeling that it is impossible to provide complete safety and simply decide to "take their chances" and go on with normal decision making and normal life. Others may decide that the only appropriate response is to drop everything else, accompany the child at every moment, and minimize any new experiences. Both strategies may provide the parent with some initial relief, but both are fraught with problems. Neither strategy is in the best interest of you or your child. Your child's life is at stake if you take unnecessary risks for the sake of normalcy or if you do not insist on his or her EpiPen being with him or her at all times. Your child's emotional health is in jeopardy if you shelter the child from every new experience or stunt his or her age-appropriate independence and growing self-esteem by your constant presence.

Making the commitment to adopt this new decision-making process is difficult whether your child has just been diagnosed or, if after years of struggling, you realize you need help in safely managing the care of your food-allergic child. I can say from experience that it is most difficult while the adjustment to this new decision-making process is being made. During this time you will be attempting to truly understand the medical realities involved with food allergies. You will need to take this medical knowledge and look at each little decision with a willingness to accept the conclusions you arrive at. It is not always easy, but as you begin to make good decisions, you will find over time that many situations come up again and again, and you will already have your answer.

Many things, like how to handle a baby-sitter or the baseball coach or lunch in the school cafeteria, will already be safely resolved. You will experience a sense of relief and confidence that comes from knowing you are doing everything you can to provide your child with a safe and normal life. Your child will begin to experience a new sense of safety and may respond with positive personality changes, becoming more outgoing or feeling less of a need to engage in troublesome behaviors such as acting out in order to feel attended to. New situations will continue to come up, and you will have to go right back to the beginning in dealing with them, as will happen each September when dealing with a new teacher or a new friend or activity. After eight years of dealing with food allergies our lives sometimes seem almost normal and care-free, but I can feel the difference in managing my two nonallergic daughters' lives. It does not strike fear in me when they receive a birthday invitation to go to an amusement park an hour away or to enjoy the spontaneity of grabbing a bite to eat at the mall while shopping. I am quick to say yes when an unexpected play date arises for them, or to enjoy the convenience of a carpool situation. We need to accept that serious food allergies make managing certain aspects of our children's lives more complicated, and we must be willing to deal with this.

Only then will you be able to see the allergy for what it is and not be paralyzed by your fears: that your child may die; that your child is different; that the carefree life you wanted for your child is now gone. After being honest with yourself and others, you will be able to really take in all the basic medical information you will need to become familiar with, and to take these facts into consideration when making decisions about your child and family. It is ironic that only after fully realizing how deep and far-reaching the implications of the food allergy are will you be able to actually minimize the effects that it does have on your family. This is the goal. The point is not to wallow in self-pity but to work through what you do feel in order to make the daily decisions that will ultimately make your child as physically and emotionally healthy as possible. You and your family in turn will reap the benefits of helping your child have the safest environment possible, the most normal childhood possible, and the least amount of anxiety necessary.

I would recommend beginning the process of educating yourself about your child's diagnosis by asking yourself the most revealing question of all, "How did I find out about my child's allergy?" I would like to answer this question myself to share with you my story. I have found listening to others' stories strangely healing and sometimes inspirational. You are not alone.

MY STORY

My son, Max, is our firstborn and simply was a delightful baby in almost every way. I am reluctant to say he was a good baby because that would imply that a baby with a lower tolerance level would have to be called a bad baby. I will say that his needs were so limited and so easily met that he was extremely easy to care for, and this made for a very happy household. A day care provider who watched him for short periods of time used to comment that it did not seem right to accept money from me to care for this happy infant. In my naïveté I was tempted to attribute his fabulous disposition to my keen and effortless skill and instinct as a mother. (I have since given birth to two daughters who have wasted no time in letting me know that skill or instinct had absolutely nothing to do with my son's behavior and disposition. If anything, the girls have led me to believe that I must surely be lacking some essential skill or instinct! But that is the topic of yet another book entirely.)

Max never had any trouble with breast milk or formula in his bottle. He progressed from rice cereal to fruits, then vegetables, meats, and finally table food. When Max was eleven months old, I rented a small cottage in a nearby beach community to experience the kind of summer vacation that I had always dreamed of. My husband's schedule did not allow for vacation time in the summer, so he made the hour-long commute before and after work to be with us. One day, I had gone for a leisurely grocery-shopping trip with Max. We picked out new summer fruits for him to try, such as peaches and plums. I also purchased a tiny jar of peanut butter. I had read somewhere that peanut products should not be given to babies until their first birthday (although it did not say why), and that date being just a couple of weeks away, I could not wait for Max to taste the food that I had practically lived on for the first ten years of my life.

Upon returning to the cottage, our bodies still sandy from our earlier visit to the beach, I prepared to sit down and feed the baby. I opened up the jar of peanut butter and decided to let Max try it first on a little plastic baby spoon. His mouth no sooner made contact with the spoon than he began howling and rubbing his eyes. Max almost never cried, so I couldn't imagine what the problem could be. I stopped feeding him and watched as his eyes became redder and redder as he rubbed and pounded his little face. All at once, giant hives appeared on his face and stomach. His neck looked as if it was swelling, getting wider and wider, and his ears became thick and bright red. Max continued to cry as I lifted him up to assess what I should do. It was then that he began projectile vomiting all over me. Waves of vomit continued to spew out of his tiny mouth, and I became extremely alarmed. I ran with him to the nearest cottage, where the occupant I had met earlier tried to calm me, as by now I was crying right along with Max. This more experienced mother of three told me that Max was probably allergic to the peanut butter but that it was *just* an allergic reaction. She suggested an over-the-counter liquid allergy medication for hives. She did not think I should take him to the hospital. I had absolutely no idea that an allergic reaction to food could be life-threatening at the time, but I did know that what she was telling me just did not fit with what I was seeing. Max was getting increasingly worse with more hives, crying, and swelling.

I returned to the lovely seaside cottage I had rented, which had no phone. Suddenly this dream vacation seemed like the worst idea I had ever had in my life. I managed to make a call from my temperamental car phone to Max's doctor's office and was told to go directly to the nearest emergency room. I frantically wrote a note to my husband, who was due to arrive any minute. He arrived just as I was jumping back into the car and must have been thoroughly confused as I told him—crying and muttering something about peanut butter—to get in and drive to the hospital. We were not sure exactly where the hospital was, so we started to drive in that general direction hoping to see signs. Only after a couple of wrong turns did we manage to pull into the emergency room parking lot. By now I was in a panic.

The staff took us in fairly quickly upon seeing my son's swollen and red body. They immediately treated him with an injection of epinephrine and a dose of liquid antihistamine. We then spent a good amount of time in the examination room so that the doctors could observe Max, who looked more like a tiny version of the Michelin Tire Man than our baby. I have bittersweet memories of this time at the hospital. Realizing that everything was under control, we were filled with such a great sense of relief that we became almost giddy at the sight of our baby careening back and forth on the gurney from the effects of the adrenaline on his body. I remember how odd it was to see our usually reserved baby jumping around like a little monkey. Since I was technically on vacation, I had my camera in Max's diaper bag. We took a picture for our well-labeled photo album of his life that, until now, had been picture-perfect.

The emergency room staff simply told us that

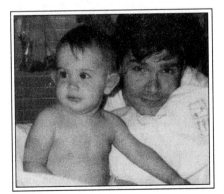

Max and father, Bill Collins

Max was obviously allergic to peanut butter and to avoid it in the future. This sounded reasonable to us, and we were glad that he was released that evening. I was so relieved that I quickly put the whole experience out of my mind. I was unaware then that peanut allergies are considered to be the most lethal, that the danger is lifelong, and that avoiding accidental exposure would be difficult. It was only as an afterthought that I even mentioned the emergency event at a well-baby visit with my son's doctor. He knew enough to immediately schedule an appointment with a pediatric allergist.

During his first visit to the allergist, Max was scratch-tested on his back to many common allergens. I became alarmed when I saw the giant red and swollen wheal that appeared where peanut had been tested, as well as all the other angry-looking wheals that appeared indicating that Max had allergies to every tree nut that the doctor chose to test him for. I started to get worried. It was at the consultation with the doctor, immediately following the results of the tests, that the seriousness of Max's allergy began to sink in. The doctor was kind and sympathetic but did not pull any punches. He explained that what my son had experienced at the beach cottage was called anaphylaxis, a general body reaction involving one or more systems of the body. We would need to be vigilant in preventing another reaction to all tree nuts as well as peanuts, as Max was at great risk, between the history of his reaction and positive skin tests, for experiencing anaphylaxis again. (Tree nuts include almonds; Brazil nuts; cashews; chestnuts; filberts, otherwise known as hazelnuts; hickory nuts; macadamia nuts; pecans; pine nuts, otherwise known as pinyon nuts; pistachios; and walnuts.) The doctor told us stories of children who hadn't lived through anaphylaxis and said he could not explain why some kids did while others did not. He did say that the way for us to increase the odds of having Max survive was by doing our best to prevent exposure; by being able to recognize a possible reaction, which could present itself in several different ways: and by always carrying injectable epinephrine with us. We were instructed to inject it at the first sign of a serious reaction and to follow the injection with a visit to the emergency room. This was a lot to digest and was rather shocking.

At the time, Max did not meet the minimum weight requirement to safely use the premeasured auto-injector of epinephrine, or EpiPenJr. We would instead need to carry glass ampules filled with epinephrine and separate injection needles. The doctor would not let us leave until we could break open the ampule, draw up the correct amount of epinephrine, and inject it into an orange. I remember that tears were rolling down my cheeks as I awkwardly injected the orange while looking over at my smiling, innocent baby. I looked at my husband, not knowing if he was feeling the confusion and sadness that I was, hoping all the while that I was misunderstanding what I had been hearing. I hoped his recollection of what had transpired was not what I had begun to understand. But what he had heard was indeed what I had heard, and he was equally shocked and hurt.

When I arrived home, I began to report the outcome of the doctor visit to my family members and close friends. They all meant well, but it was hard to find the support I needed. I was either met with pity and grave concern for Max or with casual responses indicating that my family and friends did not understand the seriousness of the allergy. Neither response was helpful. All this took place many years ago, and the Food Allergy Network was just being formed. Little if any information was available, and food allergy awareness was extremely low.

My response to this lack of information and support was to turn off my worry as much as possible. I lacked the necessary tools to deal with my son's allergy effectively. I let people know about the allergy, but I didn't follow through nearly as much as I should have. I was not making decisions with Max's allergy in mind. I simply continued living the way we had planned. I even continued with vacation plans that, in retrospect, put my son at risk, due to the lack of emergency treatment available. As a result of not being honest with myself I experienced what I call panic attacks, which would sneak up on me at unpredictable times. The worry was not gone, it was just hidden from my everyday thoughts. It would surprise me and come to me in full force, refusing to be ignored. Our family may have been enjoying vacations and daily life without restrictions, but the high price was the unnecessary risk to my son's life and an undercurrent of anxiety that affected every aspect of our life.

A turning point came three years later when Max was retested for the allergy to peanuts and many additional tree nuts. He was four years old, and his testing positive for all of them hit me like a ton of bricks. I had not known it consciously, but I had begun to believe out of necessity that he would somehow grow out of the allergies or that something would change. When neither of these things happened, I knew it was me who needed to make some changes.

My son's allergist hooked me up with the Food Allergy Network, which was now running at full steam, and I began to see the light at the end of the tunnel. I had made a friend locally whose child also suffered from multiple allergies. We often felt the same way about things and I began to feel supported enough to start becoming educated and making the necessary changes in my thoughts and actions.

I decided to conduct research, searching internationally for every bit of information on food allergies and anaphylaxis ever written. After learning about the physiology of anaphylaxis, I could not help but be intrigued by the many different responses of families to living with the management of a child's food allergies. I was phoned by one parent seeking state-provided respite care from the demands of caring for a child with a peanut allergy, while another parent reported that she did not regularly carry an EpiPen. As a family therapist, I could quickly see the pitfalls that this unique health concern posed to families. I developed a questionnaire for parents of food-allergic children that asked both factual and family dynamics questions. I was surprised by the attention and detail parents gave to my lengthy survey. In an era highlighted by a general lack of free time, I was amazed at the time people took to offer additional information, support for my work, and even expressions of thanks. I was compelled to follow up with phone interviews with parents all over the country. I knew I had tapped into an area that I needed to do justice to. And so the idea for this book was born.

Armed with all the knowledge I could obtain through research and great ideas about managing food allergies gleaned from the parents I had spoken to, I first put my efforts into making my own child as safe and happy as possible. I do not even like to write this for fear of tempting fate, but Max has remained reaction-free since his initial reaction. This has to be attributed to massive amounts of education, cooperation from his school and many caregivers, special prayers, and a little luck. Feeling confident that I am doing all that I can do for my son, and having gained the support from friends to deal with the anxiety about matters that are out of my control, I went forward with trying to help other parents. I did not want parents of newly diagnosed children to feel isolated and lost as I had. I wanted to at least provide them with a map of the process they would undergo. I also wanted parents of children diagnosed years ago to make sense of what they have been through and continue to make their lives physically and emotionally healthier.

2

FOOD ALLERGY
BASICS

————— ~ —————

Much OF THE INFORMATION contained in this chapter
has been compiled from the most recent materials available from
the Food Allergy Network, and I thank them again for sharing this
information with us. Since medical discoveries are constantly
being made, I urge the reader to become a member of this nonprofit
organization. For a nominal fee you will receive a bimonthly newsletter that will keep you abreast of the most up-to-date medical
information available.

If you are feeling overwhelmed by the prospect of keeping
your food-allergic child safe on a moment-to-moment basis, making the effort to fully understand the physiology of food allergies
may seem like a waste of energy. You may be more interested in
what to do about the first birthday party your food-allergic child

has been invited to than learning more about mast cells and immunoglobulin E.

Medical terminology can be intimidating. Still, it is vital that you have a full understanding of what is physically happening during a reaction. This information is important for making good decisions about daily life. It also helps when you have to communicate your child's needs to others. You are then able to reinforce your requests with specific medical facts and quickly correct any mistaken beliefs people have about allergies.

Many people are confused about the issue of food allergies. Part of the reason may be due to semantics. One doctor explained it this way: "It is as if there are not enough words in the English language to accurately discuss allergies." We tend to identify all adverse reactions to food as *allergies*, when in fact this is not the case.

Reactions to food can be allergic or nonallergic. Allergic reactions involve the immune system, while nonallergic reactions do not. *Food intolerance* is a more accurate term for a nonallergic reaction. True allergic reactions can usually be distinguished from food intolerance by means of the symptoms, but occasionally the reactions may appear quite similar. Yet, the causes of the resulting reactions are clearly different. A skilled allergist can usually make the distinction between a true allergy and a food intolerance based on the patient's reaction history and skin and blood tests.

A nonallergic reaction is caused by mechanisms in the gastrointestinal (GI) tract that do not involve the immune system. For example, a person who has an intolerance to milk may be lactose-intolerant. This means the individual lacks a necessary enzyme in the GI tract that would otherwise break down the lactose, or milk protein. The result may be GI symptoms such as abdominal cramps and diarrhea.

A complete account of what actually happens during a true allergic reaction is not yet known or agreed upon by the medical profession. While there seems to be agreement that the immune system is involved in an allergic reaction, there is still disagreement regarding which elements of the immune system are involved.

THE IMMUNE SYSTEM RESPONSE

The current theory is that during an allergic reaction the immune system produces IgE, or immunoglobulin E, an antibody to the particular food protein the body finds to be offensive. The IgE antibodies then attach themselves to special cells in the body called mast cells, where they can stay for a long period of time without any harmful effects. However, in a subsequent exposure to this same food protein, the immune system recognizes the protein, and its previously sensitized mast cells "lock" onto the offending food protein and trigger a response. This response is the release of histamine and other inflammatory chemicals acting as mediators. It is actually the histamine and other chemicals that result in symptoms being experienced in the GI tract and systemically throughout the rest of the body. One possible explanation for the immune system response is that a case of mistaken identity is occurring. The body may erroneously identify the otherwise harmless food protein as a dangerous invader, such as a virus, and the flood of histamines is released in an effort to rid the body of what it perceives as an unwelcome intruder. This overreaction of the immune system to a nonexistent enemy only manages to wreak havoc on the body as a flood of inflammatory chemicals is manufactured and delivered unnecessarily.

In this way, an individual with a true allergy to milk may experience cramps and diarrhea, but the cause of the reaction is quite different from that in the individual experiencing GI symptoms from a lactose intolerance. The potential consequences for the truly allergic individual are also much more serious, and in some cases may result in death.

SYMPTOMS OF AN ALLERGIC REACTION

The flood of histamine and other chemicals released during an allergic reaction exerts its effects on the various organ systems such as the skin, the respiratory system, the gastrointestinal tract, and the cardiovascular system. Symptoms may include one or more of the following:

> Feeling of anxiety or dread
>
> Redness of skin and/or hives
>
> Warmth and swelling of skin
>
> Itching and/or swelling of lips, throat, and tongue
>
> Itchy eyes, sneezing, coughing, hoarseness
>
> Wheezing
>
> Chest and throat tightness
>
> Nausea, vomiting, abdominal cramps, diarrhea
>
> Shortness of breath
>
> Increased heart rate
>
> Loss of consciousness due to rapid and severe drop in blood pressure

Although many people say the neurological symptom of a "feeling of dread" is experienced at the time of exposure to an offending food, physical symptoms may occur in as little as two minutes or as long as two hours after ingestion.

The most serious allergic reaction is called *anaphylaxis*. It is sometimes called a "general body reaction" or "general shock" and refers to one or more body systems experiencing symptoms during one reaction. Left untreated or undertreated, anaphylaxis can result in death.

Each reaction in an allergic individual can vary in its onset, symptoms, and severity. There is no way to predict how a reaction will progress, although it is most common for the first symptoms to appear within thirty minutes of exposure with the reaction worsening over the next ninety minutes. Some reactions diminish as soon as medication is administered. Others escalate from mild symptoms to full-blown anaphylaxis within minutes or in less common cases there can be a lag time of up to two hours before symptoms even begin to develop. Still others improve with medication only to come back within minutes or hours. This second flare-up is called a biphasic reaction and may be more life-threatening because it can catch the individual off guard and can be less responsive to treatment than the first reaction. It is critical to remain at the emergency room for at least three to four hours after the resolution of a serious reaction, even if the hospital staff says you can leave.

Anaphylaxis can also be induced by adverse reactions to bee and wasp venom, exercise, latex rubber, and medications such as penicillin, as well as unknown causes, referred to as idiopathic. It is believed that more children die from food-related anaphylaxis than from bee stings each year. It is also many allergists' experience that food-induced reactions are the major cause of anaphylaxis.

According to the Food Allergy Network, the eight foods that account for more than 90 percent of all allergic reactions in children are milk, eggs, peanuts, tree nuts, fish, shellfish, soy, and wheat. A study published in the *Journal of Allergy and Clinical Immunology* estimated that 1.1 percent of the population, or close to three million Americans, are affected by a peanut or tree-nut allergy. However, many other foods also cause allergic reactions. Although most children outgrow many of their food allergies, an allergy to peanuts, tree nuts, or seafood is usually considered lifelong.

The amount of food necessary to cause an allergic reaction varies from individual to individual. John Yunginger, M.D., concluded in a 1988 study that fatal reactions can be induced by as little as 1 milligram of food. For many food-allergic individuals, the offending food does not even need to be ingested to produce an anaphylactic reaction. There are reports of anaphylactic reactions occurring as the result of kisses on the skin or lips. A five-year-old girl experienced an anaphylactic reaction when a small amount of nut entered her thumb through a prick by a pointy acorn as she was feeding squirrels in the park. A nine-year-old boy had a reaction from merely touching a peanut butter bird feeder and later wiping his eye. Another child, an eight-year-old girl, succumbed to the mere vapors of garbanzo beans, also known as chickpeas, cooking on the stove. She experienced an anaphylactic reaction without ever touching, or otherwise ingesting, the beans. She was brought to an area hospital but died three days later. Yet another individual suffered a full-blown anaphylactic reaction and died from simply inhaling the fumes of a steaming platter of shrimp passing by her restaurant table.

TREATMENT

A great deal of research is currently being conducted to find a cure for food allergies. This was not the case less than a decade ago. Strides are being made fairly quickly to identify the specific portions of food allergens that cause allergic reactions, which may be used to develop strategies for treating food allergies. Promising studies are being conducted in which researchers are striving for ways to essentially "turn off" the allergic response for specific foods. Researchers are also working on anti-IgE antibodies, such that these antibodies interfere with IgE-mediated responses and appear to "turn off" the antibodies responsible for an allergic reaction to any food. This is a hopeful time for food-allergy sufferers.

But for now, there is no cure for food allergies, and the only preventive treatment is strict food avoidance. The standard treatment for a food-allergic reaction is the injection of epinephrine, the frontline drug used in anaphylactic reactions. It is available in premeasured automatic injectors designed for self-injection and given different pharmaceutical trademarked names such as EpiPen, EpiPenJr. (for children), and Ana-Kit. New products are now being considered by the Food and Drug Administration and are likely to make it to market fairly soon. For simplicity's sake I will refer to the auto-injector of epinephrine as an "EpiPen."

The assessment of reactions is sometimes obvious and sometimes difficult. The same individual may have a different reaction each time he or she is exposed to the same allergen. The symptoms may vary as well as the way the symptoms present themselves. The Food Allergy Network reports that one reaction may appear mild at first and gradually become severe. Another may start out mild and resolve itself. Still another may suddenly appear and become instantly severe. Given the unpredictable nature of allergic reactions and severity of the symptoms, all reactions must be taken seriously.

Treatment involves administering the EpiPen to the outer thigh area, followed by a dose of oral antihistamine. Immediate transportation to the nearest hospital emergency room is necessary. There, the patient may require further lifesaving treatment. If the reaction subsides, the individual should remain for three hours for observation in case of a biphasic reaction. The EpiPen is effective for only fifteen to twenty minutes, and its purpose is to give the individual time to reach the emergency room, where additional treatment may be needed. If transport time to the emergency room exceeds fifteen to twenty minutes and the patient's symptoms are worsening, there may be the need to administer an additional EpiPen. If the patient is in a remote location or experiences a delay in transport, one additional EpiPen may be required for each fifteen- to twenty-minute time period that passes. The decision to administer a second EpiPen should also be based on the severity of the symptom experienced regardless of the passage of time. For instance, if fifteen to twenty minutes has not passed, but the patient's symptoms have worsened, a second EpiPen may need to be administered.

Even if it is unnecessary, receiving an EpiPen injection should not have serious consequences. According to the Physician Insert of the EpiPen, accidental injection of the EpiPen into the hands and feet may result in loss of blood flow to the affected area and should be avoided. If there is accidental injection into these areas, the patient should go immediately to the nearest emergency room for treatment. When an injection and a trip to the hospital turn out to have been unnecessary, it is merely an uncomfortable nuisance. Not receiving an injection and not going to the hospital when necessary may result in death. It is always wiser to err on the side of caution.

Allergies on the Rise

As mentioned earlier, food allergies are thought to affect 5 percent of children. Although firm data are not yet available, doctors who investigate food allergies believe the frequency of food-induced anaphylactic reactions has risen over the past several years and will continue to rise. One explanation for the expected rise is the increased use of protein additives in commercially prepared foods. Another possible explanation is the increased use of certain asthma inhalers, which may produce a state of dependence with a heightened susceptibility to bronchospasm. The investigation continues into other possible explanations for the alarming rise in food allergies.

It should be noted that there may be a link between asthma and food allergies. According to recent studies, the complications associated with asthma make an allergic reaction even more life threatening. This is important to remember when planning how to quickly recognize and aggressively treat an anaphylactic reaction. In a study by Mendelson, Rosen, and Sampson of fatal and near-fatal anaphylactic reactions, published in 1992 in the *New England Journal of Medicine,* all thirteen cases involved children with asthma. In twelve of those children, the asthma was well controlled. In my own informal survey of parents of food-allergic children, an overwhelming majority reported that their child also suffered from asthma (although my son does not). Even so, asthma was not a problem for some children in the informal survey. To learn more about caring for a child with asthma, a wonderful resource is *A Parent's Guide to Asthma* by Nancy Sander.

THE RISK OF ACCIDENTAL EXPOSURE

Although strict food avoidance is prescribed for food-allergic children and is successful in theory, attempts at practicing food avoidance are often unsuccessful. In the 1992 study published in the *New England Journal of Medicine,* five of the six children who died had previously had an allergic reaction to the same food responsible for the fatal reaction. The same was true for six of the seven children who nearly died. The virtual impossibility of successful food avoidance was further shown in a 1989 follow-up study of children with an allergy to peanuts. Fifty percent of the children had accidentally ingested some form of peanuts in the year before the survey, and 75 percent had done so within the preceding five years.

All of the children who experienced fatal or near-fatal allergic reactions had accidentally ingested the foods responsible for the reactions, unbeknownst to them or their parents. Of the six children who died, three of them reacted to peanuts, two to nuts, and one to eggs. The allergens were concealed in a cupcake, a sandwich, a hamburger roll, and, in three cases, candy.

Even when parents and children are vigilant about identifying ingredients, mistakes can happen. Sometimes a person simply does not know what is in a food and misstates the ingredients. Other errors occur when an individual has a misunderstanding of allergies, assuming that the child will experience only an upset stomach or a stuffy nose. This person may mistakenly disregard the need for accurate ingredient listings. There can also be numerous safety lapses in the process of manufacturing, storage, packaging, and serving of food products. Finally, cross-contamination can occur when offending food ingredients are used in the allergic child's own home.

Instances of accidental exposure are all too common. Be careful of:

◆ Well-meaning people who mistake the ingredients in a food

◆ People who have a misunderstanding of allergies and do not understand that a tiny amount of food can be life threatening

◆ Exposure to toddlers or children who tend to leave food on their bodies or clothing and cannot understand the concept of exposing others

◆ The presence of the offending ingredient in unlikely foods

◆ Ingredient label changes since the last time you read the label

◆ Cross-contamination in your own home on countertops or utensils and (for those with a peanut allergy) in jelly or marshmallow fluff jars

◆ Cross-contamination in the manufacturing, packaging, or storage of foods that you buy

◆ Cross-contamination of foods purchased at bakeries, restaurants, or ice cream parlors

On two occasions I found nuts in food that was supposed to be nut-free. One was in a Danish from a bakery and the other was in ice cream from an ice cream parlor. Luckily, the nuts were discovered upon visual inspection before my son had eaten them. Many parents of food-allergic children can relate similar experiences. Bakeries, ice cream parlors, and restaurants are particularly prone to these kinds of errors.

Perhaps the most publicized example of the most serious kind of error was a multi-million dollar lawsuit that was brought against a large restaurant chain. A thirty-three-year-old woman was at the restaurant when she asked her waitress to list the ingredients of the pesto sauce. The woman was allergic to nuts, and when nuts were not among the list of ingredients, she went ahead and ordered it. When she received the dish, she asked the waitress directly if the pesto sauce had nuts in it. The waitress allegedly stated that no nuts were in the sauce when in fact it contained both pine nuts and walnuts. The woman went into anaphylactic shock and later died.

Label reading and inquiring about ingredients are essential in attempting to manage food avoidance. Parents of food-allergic children learn quickly that relying on one's own instincts in deciding when they need to read a label can be a mistake. There is an insidiousness about offending ingredients, especially peanuts. Peanuts, actually a member of the legume family, have been found on the labels of many unlikely foods, including Raisinets, plain M&M's, hot chocolate, and brown gravy. You must read *all* food ingredient labels, not just the ones where you would expect to find the offending ingredient.

CROSS-CONTAMINATION

Cross-contamination in the food production and packaging industry poses a problem for food-allergic children and adults alike. Shared equipment in food production and packaging lines can result in cross-contamination of food, especially cereals and candy. For example, manufacturers cannot guarantee the safety of a nut-free cereal or candy that is produced in the same machines used to make cereals and candy that do contain nuts. In this case, manufacturers will include a statement on the label reading "May contain peanuts."

A process called "reworking" also poses a danger for those with severe food allergies. This refers to the process by which an ice cream flavor containing nuts is produced and the base flavor is screened to make another flavor not containing nuts. For instance, a manufacturer may start with a rich base that contains ground nuts for flavor and then use this base in all other flavors, including plain vanilla. This method is used to enhance the flavor of the ice cream not containing nuts.

The danger of cross-contamination is present in school cafeterias as well as a child's own kitchen. A teenage girl who was allergic to peanuts died as a result of an anaphylactic reaction caused by cross-contamination in her kitchen. She used a knife she found on the counter that looked clean but that, unbeknownst to her, had been used to make a peanut butter sandwich and then wiped clean. She died of an anaphylactic reaction within forty-five minutes.

3

KEEPING YOUR
FAMILY
HEALTHY

─────── ∽ ───────

I T HAS BEEN SAID that living with a child who has a potentially life-threatening food sensitivity is difficult and emotionally
taxing. In my own opinion—and according to the dozens of parents I have interviewed—this is an understatement.

There are ways to ease your family's burden. Although it is difficult to accept the information available about anaphylaxis, it is
important for families to become educated. Even when you know
all the facts, there are still ambiguities about food allergies. But
living with some ambiguity is safer for your child than living with
fear of the unknown. Reliable information enables you to make
educated decisions about your child's daily life.

It is also vital to have some sort of map of what lies ahead.
This chapter, in particular, covers the family dynamics and problems

that you may face. Although managing the care of a child with a serious food allergy is precarious, at least the experience can be made more predictable. Your goal is to normalize experiences, be better able to put experiences and feelings into perspective, and not feel so isolated.

Every child is different, every child's allergies different, every family different, and every child's environment different. Yet, families describe remarkably similar experiences and emotions associated with keeping their child safe. The question becomes how your family will react to what lies ahead.

WHERE TO BEGIN— SAFETY IN THE HOME

I am frequently contacted by parents with newly diagnosed food-allergic children, and first and foremost they want to know how to make their home safe. What should or shouldn't the child eat? They seem to be hoping that I will have the one piece of information that will make everything safe. I wish I did. Learning to manage this kind of allergy is a process that takes time.

After reading about Food Allergy Basics in chapter 1, you have the foundation upon which to build further knowledge that is specific to your child and the body of knowledge you will accumulate about the offending food item(s). You must begin by reading the label of every food item brought into your home. This is where you need to *turn off your common sense* regarding which items might contain the offending ingredient. Experience will show you that the allergen will turn up in all kinds of unlikely places. The only action you can take is to systematically check all labels in your home and check them *regularly,* because they *do* change. In order to find out which food products you will need to eliminate from your child's diet, you will need to learn all the possible names for the offending food(s) so that you know what you are looking for on these labels. The Food Allergy Network has inexpensive ingredient cards available that list all the possible names to look for specific to each common food allergen. I highly recommend this, as there are some words used on labels that you may not associate with the particular food you are trying to avoid. For example, the term *casein* indicates the presence of milk protein, and *pinyon* and *pignolia nut* are other words for pine nuts.

When considering which foods to eliminate based on the chance of cross-contamination, you will need to *reactivate your common sense* and use it constantly. You need to imagine the production of foods and consider the possibility that cross-contamination can occur in raw material containers, processing machinery, packaging machinery, and display cases. Many times a label will be free of an allergen, but your common sense will tell you that the probability of cross-contamination is high. Perhaps the manufacturer has not yet been brought up to speed on this danger or has not gone public with the risk. For instance, my common sense told me that granola bars without nuts listed on the label were not the best choice for my son when there were five other varieties of nut-containing granola bars available from the same manufacturer. Years later, this risk was acknowledged when manufacturers reported that there is cross-contamination on the production lines, due partly to the gooeyness of the product. Effective cleaning of production lines is not easily achieved. I also use my common sense in not allowing my son to eat a giant gourmet nut-free cookie when it is merchandised in a beautiful wicker basket right next to peanut butter cookies. If the cookie was not contaminated in the basket, it may have been contaminated in the "gourmet" mixing bowl. Consider it a red flag when you read "gourmet" or "secret sauce" on a product. The more upscale the product, the more likely it is that nuts are an ingredient, even if it is not obvious to the eye. For peanut- or nut-allergic children, baked goods and

Asian food items are the top two cross-contamination risks. Follow the rule, and when in doubt, skip the food! This applies to products with or without labels. The Food Allergy Network also lists types of food that you should be especially careful of on their ingredient cards.

There is some debate over whether the offending food item(s) should be eliminated from your household entirely. Many parents feel that their child must learn to coexist with the offending food item(s), so the process may as well start at home. This is a good point, but one must be ever-vigilant of accidents involving cross-contamination of utensils, counters, and other surfaces. I have even heard of a peanut butter sandwich made for a nonallergic sibling's lunch making its way into a peanut-allergic child's lunch box. This is not an unlikely occurrence when you consider that a parent is usually making several children's lunches five mornings per week in a sometimes hectic environment.

When considering elimination of the food item from the home, a parent should consider the ages of the members of the household and the level of worry they can live with. Since we have three young children, we have decided that for now we will eliminate any obvious peanut and tree-nut products from our home. Perhaps when all members of the household reach a responsible age and can be counted on to understand safe food preparation and handling, we will reconsider this decision. A parent should also consider how easy or healthy it would be for the other members of the family to live without the offending food. For example, it is easy for us to do without peanut and tree-nut products, as there are many other healthy food alternatives available to us. But if milk or eggs were the offending food, it would not be healthy or desirable for siblings and even parents to live without them. In this case, systems of safely storing, using, and disposing of the offending food must be developed and strictly adhered to.

Having some sort of plan in the kitchen becomes very important, especially in those families where the child is allergic to foods that are hard to avoid, such as egg, wheat, and milk. Foods deemed safe for the child may be kept in a separate area of the kitchen, such as a designated cabinet shelf and refrigerator shelf, physically separated from all foods that would be unsafe for the child. The safe food could even be labeled with some sort of bright sticker. This would minimize the risk that any family member or caregiver might give an unsafe food to the child. Food preparation areas could be designated as safe or unsafe as well. For example, one cutting board could be reserved for use when preparing food for the food-allergic child to minimize the risk of cross-contaminating the safe food. A separate counter or board, as well as separate utensils, may be utilized when preparing unsafe foods such as a peanut butter and jelly sandwich for other family members. There should be a procedure for washing the area and utensils with a brush or sponge that will not be used on the food-allergic child's utensils, dishes, or table surface. Hand washing followed by drying with a disposable paper towel should also be done by anyone preparing an unsafe food. A practice of using only disposable plates and utensils when preparing and eating unsafe foods may work well in minimizing the risk of cross-contamination in the kitchen. Be careful of cross-contamination in other people's homes, as well. For instance, be wary of having a neighbor prepare a seemingly safe jelly sandwich for your peanut-allergic child, as chances are there is peanut product in the jelly jar. In our case, extended family members keep a separate jar of jelly for my son brightly labeled and in a remote corner of their refrigerator.

An emergency kit with the EpiPen, if prescribed, and a liquid antihistamine should always be in an easily accessible place in case of an emergency. All family members should be trained in dialing 911. Have a plan. It is also a good idea for your child to wear some sort of medical emergency identification jewelry. You may not feel the need to do this with a young child who is always with someone who is aware of the allergy, but it is helpful to emergency technicians in the event of an emergency. It is also good for young children to become accustomed to wearing one at an early age so they are used to it when they do venture out in the world. The phone numbers of several medical emergency identification jewelry companies are listed in the Resource Guide of this book.

EATING OUT

When it comes to eating away from home at restaurants and other homes, I am also very conservative. Due to the uneducated responses we have experienced when we have eaten out, and our basic knowledge of what restaurant kitchens look like and how they function, we are not very comfortable with the option of eating out. When you must eat out, let the waitstaff, and preferably the manager or the cook, know of your child's food allergy. Tell them which food(s) your child must avoid and explain the danger of even the tiniest trace of cross-contamination. Ask them to recommend which item would be safest. But be prepared. Sometimes you will be met by complete misunderstanding at best and plain rudeness at worst. Sometimes the staff does not want to accept responsibility for claiming a food is safe. Where does this leave your child? If you have managed to have a good and safe dining experience at a few restaurants, I would stick to them, and avoid experimenting when it comes to restaurants. *Do not enter an eating establishment without your child's emergency medication kit.*

TRAVELING

The extent to which you feel comfortable traveling with your food-allergic child is a particularly personal one. Parents have varied opinions and comfort levels when it comes to traveling. I know some who have taken transatlantic flights and traveled around

Europe for the summer without a great deal of anxiety, and others who would not consider flying on a shuttle to the nearest city for a weekend. Some feel comfortable spending time in remote locations with a dozen EpiPens in tow to buy them time to get to the nearest emergency room. Others would not consider locations that are not within a minute's drive from the nearest hospital. I know I am not comfortable with the idea of a cruise, for instance, because of having to rely on the food provided and being cut off from a real hospital.

Travel by plane, where peanuts are given out at forty thousand feet, is especially scary for peanut-allergic children and their families. The major airlines are currently debating what to do about food-allergic passengers and are trying to develop some standardized rules to govern the airline industry. In 1998, the Department of Transportation issued a statement acknowledging that food allergies are a medical condition under the Air Carrier Access Act and can be life threatening. It called for actions to be taken to protect these passengers by making certain accommodations. It recommended a "buffer zone" that would consist of at least one row ahead and behind the passenger to receive a non-peanut snack. Although it was only the first step in providing safety to food-allergic passengers, this directive was later rescinded for lack of medical information about peanut allergies. This effort to work with airlines is just one of the many causes that the Food Allergy Network is engaged in.

Whatever your mode of transportation or ultimate destination, being prepared is always your best bet. Bring a small cooler of safe food and supplies for your child to eat along the way. Restock it and carry it with you for the duration of your trip so that when in doubt, your child will not have to skip eating or take risks in unfamiliar territory. Try to secure accommodations that will provide you with kitchen appliances such as a refrigerator or even a full kitchen if possible. Even if you do not like to cook on vacation (like me), you can prepare a few simple dishes that your child will safely enjoy. We consider this a necessary compromise and talk about it openly with our child. "Yes, we may enjoy this particular vacation, but for all of us to have a good and safe time you will probably need to eat a bunch of boring sandwiches that I will provide." When faced with this sacrifice, our child considers it a small price to pay, and I think he enjoys the comfort of knowing that his food is safe.

We had the most wonderful experience at Walt Disney World in Orlando, Florida. On the recommendation of a friend, we spoke to Guest Services by phone well before our arrival. It was a pleasant surprise to learn that they were well aware of the dangers of food allergies, and that they already had a protocol in place if I would be willing to make restaurant reservations ahead of time. We were contacted by the head of Food Services, who helped us iron out our itinerary in all the theme parks and pick restaurants for lunch and dinner. It was sometimes difficult to stick to the itinerary, but it was well worth it. We made reservations, and my son's needs were made known to the head chef of each restaurant. Upon our arrival at each restaurant we were met by the chef to discuss the safety of the meal he or she was planning to provide. One chef at the prestigious Grand Floridian even adapted the entire character dinner buffet to provide my son with a safe dining experience. I have neither heard of nor experienced such service before or since our trip to Disney World. They say Disney World is a place where dreams come true, and this was certainly true for me and my family!

LIVING WITH STRESS

Stress City

The foremost emotion associated with food allergies is stress, which can manifest itself in a number of different ways. Fear, responsibility, guilt, and a sense of loss can take their toll on the parents of a food-allergic child. Stress will come in different forms and at different levels. It's as if you're living in Stress City. The key is to identify and manage the times of high stress—for your well-being and your child's.

The stress probably began when your child experienced a disturbing food-induced anaphylactic reaction and ended up in an emergency room. If you were fortunate, you were referred to an allergist who specializes in children and who took a detailed history and conducted a series of tests to identify the offending foods. Many families report that their child experienced troubling symptoms for some time before they were able to find a doctor who made the proper diagnosis.

This period of time associated with experiencing the initial food-allergic reactions, positive test results, and diagnosis is one of high stress. Families are naturally frightened and confused. The newness of seeking further information about food allergies, informing others, and managing food avoidance is overwhelming.

In my case, a sympathetic and caring doctor diagnosed my son's allergies to peanuts and tree nuts. I appreciated his honesty and directness. He successfully communicated the serious nature of the risk, which helped me begin to consider realistically what actions we as parents would need to take in order to ensure the safety of our child. But this awareness of our duties as parents did not come all at once or quickly enough.

At that time I was told the medical facts. I did not realize that I had stepped onto a never-ending, exhausting merry-go-round. At first there was fear of the unknown, as I was unaware of the impact of this diagnosis.

The wheels started moving slowly, and my many questions were answered in bits and pieces. Each time there was a new realization—of just how difficult living with the risk of anaphylaxis would be, how deeply it would affect many aspects of our lives, and how little support there is—the fear intensified.

Making Fear Your Friend

I soon realized that the fear I felt wasn't all bad. Fear actually has a role in the process of managing food allergies. I found that a reasonable amount of fear could help me make good decisions about daily living. This fear, coupled with age-appropriate knowledge, also helps my son make wise decisions. Although fear should not be the only factor considered when making decisions about daily living, it can help.

One day my son was playing outside with a neighbor in my full view. The neighbor's parents called to ask me if Max could go with them to run an errand. My level of fear escalated and signaled to me that it was probably not a good idea, since this neighbor had not been trained to recognize and treat anaphylactic reactions. Another example: When Max was in kindergarten, the teacher tried to serve him an oatmeal cookie that had never been served for a snack before. Max asked the teacher about the ingredients, and after looking at its strange appearance rather discriminately, he opted to have one of his own "safe" snacks that were available to him. Fear is always present to some degree, but when it escalates, a parent or child must try not to dismiss it. Instead, listen to the fear, and act on what it is trying to tell you.

Responsibility

Many parents are worn down by the constant vigilance necessary to prevent a "theoretically preventable" reaction. If an accidental reaction occurs even while the child is in the care of another trusted individual, parents hold themselves responsible for the decisions that led to the inadvertent exposure.

We need to be thinking ahead, checking ingredients, and remembering to bring the EpiPen day in and day out. We are responsible for communicating as best we can our child's often misunderstood needs to others. Our child's life is at stake. No one is perfect, and everyone has a bad day occasionally. We as parents sometimes feel we cannot afford to be human.

Guilt

Guilt is another common and normal reaction. Guilt is experienced when an accidental reaction occurs. Some mothers feel guilty about somehow having contributed to their child's condition by eating certain foods while pregnant and nursing. Still others feel guilty because they did not nurse their children and somehow feel the allergy might have been avoided if they had.

Guilt can also haunt us when we allow our child to be involved in an activity that we later realize put our child at an unacceptable level of risk. Some parents may even feel guilty for being preoccupied with food allergies, especially when their child may look and act perfectly healthy.

Sense of Loss

Many parents of food-allergic children feel a sense of loss. Some feel it all at once when they realize that their child is not entirely "normal" or that there exists a serious health concern. Others report their heart breaking for their child at the small realizations made little by little. The child is robbed of a carefree childhood and instead must be careful and responsible before his or her time.

The diagnosis of a food allergy alters a child's life. Vacation choices may be limited because of food concerns and lack of medical facilities. Food-allergic children can never be carefree at a birthday party, restaurant, or holiday celebration—all valued experiences in our culture. The simple act of your child walking out the door without a needle ready to inject lifesaving medication is but a memory. These losses, taken individually, may seem small, but put together they are life altering. You, as well as your child, should give yourself permission to feel these losses and grieve.

Lack of Support

The simple act of receiving support could alleviate much of our stress. Unfortunately, an overwhelming majority of parents who responded to an informal survey reported a lack of support and understanding from extended family members, friends, neighbors, and schools.

The lack of support from extended family seems to be the most hurtful and difficult for parents of food-allergic children. We expect a close family member, such as a grandparent, to understand the seriousness of the situation. When this is not the case, there is emotional hurt as well as the knowledge that the child may be at a higher risk for experiencing an anaphylactic reaction when in the grandparent's presence. You feel let down by someone who could help to ease your burden. This may necessitate some hard decisions about letting your child spend time with the grandparent, or any person whose lack of understanding puts your child at risk.

Because of their own uninformed view of allergies, other people who come in contact with your child may not grasp the severity of the situation. Some people can't believe that a wholesome food could be deadly. Many people do not understand that a tiny amount of offending food can be life threatening. This leads to the mistaken belief that "he can taste a little."

One allergist described in a newspaper a tragic experience that one of his patients endured as she tried to raise awareness of food allergies. He told of a mother who was explaining her child's allergy to the hostess of a birthday party. The hostess assured the mother that the child would not be given any offending foods. Another adult helping with the party gave the peanut-allergic child a peanut butter cookie, which the child first refused. Upon her insistence, the child ate the cookie and was dead in thirty minutes. Celebrations centered around food are understandably stressful for parents of food-allergic children.

Holiday Difficulties

Holidays are especially stressful, according to many parents I have spoken with. Food is an integral part of many holiday celebrations, presenting added risk to the child with food allergies. There is also increased risk as children may be in the company of a greater number of people who do not understand food allergies. New foods may also be present, which further increases the risk to the child. Some parents of food-allergic children have said that holidays are especially difficult because extended family members take pride in their cooking, especially ethnic cooking, and it is offensive to them if the child with food allergies does not partake of the food.

Smooth Sailing

Despite the challenges and stressful times, there will be periods of smooth sailing, usually when you and others around your food-allergic child possess the knowledge necessary to create a safe and stable environment. For families surrounded by a supportive community, these periods may occur often and be long-lasting.

Coping with Stress

Living in Stress City can be dizzying. This figure illustrates what the experience of managing severe food allergies in your child might be like.

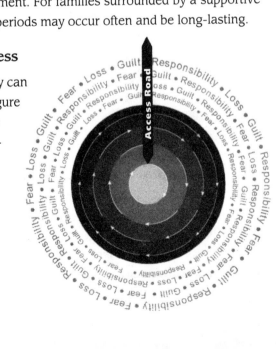

Once your child is diagnosed as having true food allergies and being at risk for experiencing a food-induced anaphylactic reaction, you are involuntarily shoved onto the circular path. Once on, if your child has an allergy that is considered lifelong, there is no way off. Each circle represents a level of stress comprised of fear, responsibility, guilt, loss, and any other emotion parents may encounter in their experience. The smallest circle represents the lowest level of stress, and the stress level rises in increments with each larger circle. Any person or situation you interact with can act as the access ramp leading you out to a circle of higher stress or in to an inner circle of lower stress, depending on the person's response to your concerns or the risk inherent in the situation.

Other than using the access road to reach the various stress levels, movement on the circles is clockwise and constant. Parents can never stop being careful, and this perpetual movement around the circles represents an endless state of vigilance. The speed of travel on the circles matches the stress level: low in the smaller circles and high in the larger circles. When situations are such that stress levels are low, we can plug along slowly on the smallest circle, in complete control of our movement. On the other hand, we may feel out of control as we are going further at higher speeds struggling to maintain control. The stress levels might change at a rapid pace during a normal day or remain the same for long periods of time. Either way, the constant movement is exhausting.

A family's response to living in Stress City can vary, depending on factors such as the amount of support received within the family and from the community. Your child's disposition, the severity of his or her allergies, and perceived level of safety available in the community may play a part. Also, a parent's ability to cope influences how he or she responds. Dysfunctional family patterns in a parent's family of origin may leave some parents with compromised coping skills. It takes an enormous amount of inner strength to manage stress, communicate with others about something "unpleasant," and deal constructively with resistance.

Seesaw Reaction

Keeping your food-allergic child physically safe and emotionally healthy can be the greatest of all balancing acts. It is as if we are standing in the middle of a seesaw, adjusting each foot to provide perfect balance. We have to work constantly to prevent either side from crashing to the ground.

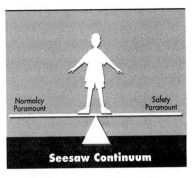

Normalcy Paramount   Safety Paramount

Seesaw Continuum

There are times when we must travel to one end or the other of the seesaw, depending on which weighty matter is threatening our child's physical safety or normal development. Many families feel stuck at one end because something has forced them to take an extreme position.

Take the example of a family that stresses normalcy above all else. Their five-year-old food-allergic girl is invited to a neighbor's house for a play date without her parent. The parent who is determined for her child to have a "normal" life may consider this part of the normal childhood experience. She may believe it is an all-or-nothing proposition: either the child participates in play with no restrictions or she does not play with others at all. In this example, the parent allows the girl to go, without telling the other family about the child's food allergies. The child is simply told not to eat anything.

As we know, this poses a risk. The time between exposure and onset of symptoms can be hours. There is also always the chance of accidental exposure (and this risk of exposure increases when the other family is not aware of the situation). The parent rationalizes, "Nothing bad is going to happen today" or "She's so close to home." The parents do not want the child to feel "different." Plus, they dread conversations about their child's allergy.

The parents who feel forced to provide normalcy above all else run an increased risk of accidental exposure, followed by an allergic reaction that may not be recognized or treated quickly enough.

On the other hand, a parent who stresses physical safety above all else might never allow his or her child to go to a neighbor's. This parent might also consider it an all-or-nothing proposition. The child would not be allowed to go to the play date because the parents may be stuck in fear. They worry that another child could expose their child. Or maybe they don't trust the playmate's parent or feel he or she doesn't have the ability to understand the needs of their child. Because any one of these fears may be perfectly justified, this parent feels that sheltering the child is best.

This level of protection may be necessary for a young child who is completely dependent on the parent. But as the sheltered child grows older, the child's emotional needs may be compromised. The normal development process may be in jeopardy. A parent who makes physical safety paramount runs the risk of the food-allergic child developing behavior problems or having a fear of separation from the parents.

BALANCING PHYSICAL SAFETY AND NORMALCY

Food-allergic children benefit most from parents who believe that physical safety is vital but who also understand that providing for normal development is important. This is most feasible when a parent has meaningful support from the extended family, a friend, a fellow parent of a food-allergic child, and the community, including schools and neighbors.

The goal is to consider any situation facing the child and family and weigh the potential benefits and risks. In the case of the play date, the parent should consider the maturity of his or her own child, the child's desire to participate, the environment of the other child's home, and how many other children will be present. The final decision should be based on the other adult's *willingness* and *capability* to manage food avoidance, recognize symptoms, and administer treatment if necessary.

You may decide the risk is too great for any one of the above factors. Or you may decide that this excursion is within safety limits and worth pursuing. Your child should understand his or her choices. If the play date is allowed, the other family will need to be educated about the food allergy and the proper use of the EpiPen. Because anaphylaxis itself involves a loss of control, your child should share the decision as to who will be told about it and how it should take place. This will help keep your child's self-esteem intact as well. Even young children have wonderful ideas on how to go about educating others about food allergies. It can also be very effective when a child illustrates the use of the EpiPen. If a child can deal with this situation, adults feel they can surely give it a try. This involvement of the child also helps him or her not to feel "talked about" in a self-conscious way.

It is wise to get a sense of the other parents' willingness to become educated about food allergies before the specifics are discussed, so as not to disappoint your child unnecessarily. The entire "other" family should be involved in the discussion, as any family member's ignorance could put the child at risk. The discussion with the other family needs to be clear and direct while communicating the manageability of the allergy.

It is also useful to allow the family to view a pertinent video such as "It Only Takes One Bite," available from the Food Allergy Network in Fairfax, Virginia, before the actual discussion. This gives the family time to digest the information, provides a context for the discussion, and will usually lead the family to develop some educated questions to ask. Always ask the family after they have all the information if they still feel comfortable with the arrangement. It's better to find out now if the parent does not feel confident about keeping your child safe or has a fear of needles.

Young children are often very good at helping to keep a food-allergic friend safe. Remember to share important information with young friends as well. For children ages three to seven, the video "Alexander, the Elephant Who Couldn't Eat Peanuts" is a wonderful resource. It is also available from the Food Allergy Network.

Ask the family if they have any specific concerns and if there is anything you can do to make their job easier, such as supplying safe snacks or coming along for the first visit. Always end by communicating your appreciation for taking on the responsibility. After a play date, check in with the adults to evaluate how things went, and ask again if there are any new questions or concerns.

This can be a taxing and time-consuming undertaking, but you will not be doing this with every person you ever meet. You may find yourself becoming a good judge of which situations are worth this effort, based on your child's desire, your confidence in the adults involved, and the potential longevity of the arrangement. This play date situation, when repeated often, will become easier for everyone. Your child's allergy will cease to be the focus of the visit. Remember to discuss periodically how things are going and review emergency procedures.

Your child's circle of friends may be smaller than other playmates' but no less wonderful. In fact, one of the advantages to this predicament is that you will find caring friends with similarly caring and responsible parents. You will make some meaningful connections for you and your child.

HOW DO WE ACHIEVE BALANCE?

You'd think that every family affected by severe food allergies would naturally connect and gain support from one another. Unfortunately, this doesn't happen as often as it should, because families who position themselves at extreme ends of the seesaw may not be able to relate to one another.

First, there needs to be an understanding that all parents are doing the best that they can for their child. No two families face the exact same situation, and no two parents have the same response to a situation.

Each family needs to assess the reality that they alone face. For example, the extent of the child's allergies should be considered, as well as the parent's own values. School options in their area need to be examined. For instance, a parent who decides to home-school a child who has allergic reactions from the mere smell of an offending food, who lives in an area where there are no school nurses on staff, and who doubts the school system's ability to meet the child's needs given the school's limited resources, should not be criticized for a decision to home-school. Home schooling does not necessarily jeopardize normal development. It may be a challenge to our society's view of a "normal" childhood, but it can be done in ways that fulfill the child's developmental needs.

You can help other parents of food-allergic children by offering understanding and support regardless of where they fall on the seesaw. If you desire to move toward a more balanced position, seek out people who you think will understand or support you. Find out more about food allergies. Assess your coping skills and enhance them by talking with other parents or through counseling.

SUPPORTING YOUR OWN FAMILY

At the time of your child's food allergy diagnosis you may not have imagined that it would affect your entire family in so many ways.

The Marital Relationship

Marital stress is inevitable when parenting a child at risk for anaphylaxis. The fact that a food allergy is a "hidden" disability makes matters more complicated. If there were outward signs of the problem, such as a wheelchair, parents might more easily rally to a similar level of concern. But the invisible nature of the condition gives rise to an ambiguity that allows parents and family members to have different perceptions of the same problem. For some, "out of sight, out of mind" best describes the level of concern. For others, the uncertainty becomes the basis for rumination over the worst possible outcome, death. Parents can often split in their ambivalence, with one parent minimizing the need to worry while the other worries enough for the whole family. When parents experience this split, both may end up feeling alone and isolated, as neither feels understood or supported.

The spouse who feels he or she is carrying the brunt of the responsibility and anxiety can easily become resentful toward the spouse who is perceived to be less concerned about the child's food allergies. The result can be anger and frustration. The child and the hyperconcerned parent run the risk of becoming enmeshed, essentially creating a barrier between themselves and the other parent. Then it becomes difficult for the isolated parent to become more involved, which only perpetuates the vicious cycle. Sometimes counseling may help spouses break unhealthy cycles, which will benefit the marital relationship as well as the entire family.

The Father's Point of View

I wanted to include a section in this book that spoke directly to fathers. This is not to say that the rest of the book is only for mothers, but it is written from the only perspective available to me, the female one. For this task, I commissioned my husband, who was glad to contribute. After all, we have been on this journey together, yet I am always the one writing and speaking about how *we* handle this. The result is, I think, a heartfelt and practical passage that women will gain much insight from, and that will help men to finally feel understood. I suggest that both partners read it.

BY BILL COLLINS

It is important to understand that while every family handles a child with a severe food allergy differently (as mentioned earlier in this book), this is true even within the same parental unit. I have wanted, from the beginning of our awareness of Max's allergy, to make sure that our son has a normal childhood. My biggest fear is that he will be stigmatized or pigeonholed by this allergy into some less-than-terrific situations. Above all, I think a kid needs to be a kid! Please do not read into this that I am in denial about the seriousness of the situation. Nothing could be further from the truth. I am a label reader, information spreader, caregiver trainer, ever-vigilant emergency injection giver, and anxious parent too, but I hide it better than our beautiful author does.

As you make your way through this situation, you realize that there is a certain amount of notoriety that comes with this allergy. On the one hand, it is good because it brings focus to the problem when explaining it to caregivers and school officials, friends, and family, but on the other hand it can bite you in the behind if your child becomes known only as "Peanut Boy" or something similar. Even worse would be if your child began to identify himself in terms of this one small portion of his identity.

I remember when Max first began school and we met with school officials to discuss how everything would be handled, and the question of transportation and the school bus came up. As has been mentioned, there is a time after breakfast that could be a problem if any cereal has been eaten that contained undeclared nut products and perhaps could start a reaction—a remote but possible scenario. The school immediately suggested a special bus, designated for kids with special needs, for Max. I would have nothing to do with that. We refused to allow this additional burden to be placed on him. All regular school buses in our town are equipped with two-way radios, and we were adamant with the bus company that it was not outside of their normal liability to have this boy on their bus, despite his allergy. We kept insisting and eventually won. This was not the first time we had battled the mind-set of adults wanting to keep him completely separate from others as a method of dealing with his allergy, and I have taken on this aspect of the problem as my own.

Before Max was born, I had begun volunteer work with burned children at a local Boston hospital where the main focus in their recovery is a return to "normalcy." The goal is to look beyond their often horrible injuries to the child that still dwells within them. The kids have little trouble with this, and it is often the adults who must do most of the work. I have carried this idea forward in dealing with Max's allergy. I refuse to allow this allergy to define his being, and I take steps to show him and others that this is but a small aspect of a wonderful little boy who has much to offer.

True to form, Max and all his friends have been a complete inspiration. Children do not have all the baggage that adults do, and as such, they completely accept him and his "peanut-free table" at lunch. They are completely aware of his allergy and accept him for who he is. They tell their parents not to put any nut products in their lunches so that they can sit at his table, ensuring he is never alone. To them, he is just another hockey player on the rink and friend at recess. This is what I want to maintain. This is what you are up against when forming your plans with adults who don't see things as simply as children do.

We dads are guys, so naturally we deal with things from a decidedly male perspective. I am a "no problem" type of person in dealing with stress. This is not a completely male trait, but it works for me. This half of the parental unit doesn't get rattled by the same things as our author does. This half does not make giant detail-laden lists of things to do. This half does not spend time hand-wringing and sweating every aspect of a situation before it is upon him. Anxiety attacks do not affect this half. This half can cook dinner, be sensitive to someone's needs, watch three kids, and fix several broken appliances simultaneously after working all day long while the author is finishing her new book or perhaps out buying new shoes. "No problem!" This lack of outward signs of stress does not mean, however, that I am not aware of the problem or situation that affects us.

One of the things that I am involved in is aviation. I fly in a Navy T34 jet trainer and do air shows and flybys, aerobatics, and formation flying. One of the first rules within this small community of individuals is that no matter what is happening, at least sounding calm and cool and collected is a tremendous asset. You can handle it, no problem. You hear this when you are on a commercial flight and the captain comes on the intercom. Cool, calm, collected. That plane could be upside down going 800 mph missing a wing and the captain would still be pointing out landmarks of interest on the way: On the left is Buffalo . . .

I think it is important to have this outlook in this situation also. (This also contributes to normalcy.) If you sit down and think about this allergy and how many threats are out there and how they affect your child, it is mind-numbing. It would be easy to be scared to the point of complete denial or *inaction. Leaving your child's well-being behind or in the hands of another is not the answer. You can handle this coolly, calmly and with "No Problem." We are dads; it's what we do. However, you must make this known to your partner. You are fully aware of the situation, it exists, and you are prepared. This allergy is best dealt with by the parents as a team! Appear at the school as a team. Meet with caregivers as a team. I can personally tell you that our meetings seem to carry much more weight when we both are present. I don't know why, but it just does. A great deal of needless stress can be relieved by one parent knowing that the other is just as capable as he or she is in any situation. Make your feelings and plans known to each other so one doesn't feel like he or she is carrying the whole load alone.*

Preparation is key. In some situations we actually carry the "kit" (which includes safe snacks) with us to hockey and baseball games, where peanuts are literally everywhere. Max puts it in a little fanny pack and we carry it in. Yes, security looks at it and asks us about it and he explains what it is (I told you he was wonderful) and they let us in. We feel it necessary here to have it on us.

All relatives' homes have one. We have gotten used to having one nearby in case of need. In my flight suit pocket I have an emergency procedures book for dealing with major problems should they arise in the aircraft, and so we have instructions in Max's kit for administering emergency aid in a high-stress situation. I wear a parachute for the same reason: preparation! If the worst happens, I am ready! Once again it does not need to be the focus of the activity; it's a minor detail for just in case (and allows for normalcy).

We have been told that there is research being done in hopes of finding a solution to this problem, but for now, nothing exists. As a dad I have to tell you this is a mind-boggling thing to deal with, but it can be done. I am extremely proud of the way my wife has chosen to meet this challenge and even prouder of my son's courage and good humor. I actually feel somewhat lucky that we have something here that we can at least fight through constant vigilance and care, and have not been stricken with some incurable disease for which there is no hope at all. Try to keep this in mind as you try to find perspective.

SIBLINGS

Siblings of food-allergic children are often the forgotten members of the process when a child has food allergies. Some siblings experience fear that they too will experience an unpredictable allergic reaction. Very young siblings with an incomplete and faulty understanding of food allergies may feel a sense of guilt that they somehow "wished" the allergies onto the affected sibling.

Don't be surprised if your non–food-allergic children feel jealousy, anger, or even resentment. They may feel jealous of your preoccupation—real or perceived—with the affected sibling and resent the extra time and attention paid to him or her. It is true that parents may be more likely to volunteer in class or chaperone field trips for the child with food allergies. "It's not fair" is an expression often voiced by siblings. My own daughter Emily has often expressed hurt and anger over the fact that my husband or I have chaperoned virtually every field trip my son has taken (and there have been *lots* of them), while we have simply not experienced the need to do this for every one of her field trips as well. We realize that this does not seem fair. All we can do is listen to her and let her know that we understand what she is saying. When she feels heard, she is less apt to take it out on her brother in various ways. I need to be careful not to try to overcompensate by agreeing to chaperone all of her field trips also. I need to remind myself and help her to understand that my job as a mom is to be fair in providing for the particular needs of each child. One of our family's goals is for each member to feel safe. As parents we provide this for each of our three children. It just happens that this goal requires more of our time and energy for our food-allergic son than it does for our girls. On field trips our daughter receives a level of safety from her teachers and adult chaperones that is acceptable to us. This is not the case with Max's life-threatening allergy when he is off site and away from the school nurse in a new environment.

It is important to find useful alternative expressions of care and concern for siblings of food-allergic children. The needs of food-allergic children may consume more time, but the needs of other children are no less important.

Siblings of food-allergic children are also affected by the allergy in daily life. The sibling's food allergies are a factor in most family decisions. Certain foods might not be allowed in the home, and activities may be curtailed, such as attending parties and eating at restaurants. Vacation destinations could be limited as well. Older siblings may feel responsible for preventing, recognizing, and treating reactions. Recognize the ways in which the nonallergic siblings' lives are affected, and offer your understanding. Also recognize when counseling may be needed for disruptive or unhealthy behaviors.

MINIMIZING HARMFUL FAMILY DYNAMICS

You can minimize potentially harmful family dynamics by encouraging open and honest communication for the entire family. Nonallergic siblings should be included in these discussions.

All members should understand the goals of the family. Two such goals might be providing maximum safety to the food-allergic child while minimizing limitations for all family members. An awareness of family goals promotes understanding of the decisions parents will need to make. It's also important to have a forum to discuss the feelings that could cause various family members to become stuck in anger, fear, or jealousy. Open communication is healthy for any family, but the complicated issues involved in dangerous food allergies make the going more treacherous. Good communication from a very early age will mean fewer problems in adolescence.

Even so, be prepared! When communication is working and members feel safe enough to express themselves, emotions such as anger, loss, and jealousy may be voiced. Some parents are not comfortable with these feelings. Remember that they are natural feelings and are better expressed in words than acted out toward themselves or each other. Limit the inappropriate behaviors that the emotions can lead to, not the emotions themselves.

4

As Your Child Grows

―――――― ∾ ――――――

Your food-allergic child's needs will change as he or she grows and matures. Your role in his or her care will need to respond to these changes.

Birth to Age Five

The very young food-allergic child depends on you completely to prevent, recognize, and treat reactions. In these early years children are exploring their world, and they will look to you for support and encouragement as they take tiny steps toward independence. This can be difficult for some parents, who will worry that the world is an unsafe place for the food-allergic child. Do whatever is necessary to create an environment that feels "safe enough" for your child to enjoy some sense of normalcy. This may make your child's "world" smaller but no less stimulating than most.

Many parents are accused of overprotecting their food-allergic child. But during this time when the child cannot speak, read, or assert him- or herself, this vigilance is necessary. When protection becomes overprotection is difficult to assess. It will depend on the maturity and disposition of your child, the quantity and severity of the allergies, the presence of asthma or other health concerns, and the level of cooperation in your child's community.

It is important for children's developing self-esteem to have an age-appropriate level of control over their food allergies. Children can come to understand that having a food allergy is just one aspect of their lives and not the very definition of themselves. This can begin early on by making toddlers aware of the allergy and teaching them to ask permission before eating anything new and not to take food from anyone except parents or caregivers. You should make it clear that danger is involved, just as you would communicate the danger of running into the street. Teach children to ask if foods contain offending ingredients as soon as verbal skills develop. One young food-allergic child's first complete sentence was, "Does this have nuts in it?"

Young children tend to take their predicament in stride if it is communicated in a confident manner and if they are allowed to enjoy an age-appropriate amount of control. Remember, your child might never remember living any other way. One allergist told me that his patients who understood and accepted their allergies from a very young age seemed to manage them better in adolescence and were less apt to take food risks.

AGES FIVE TO ELEVEN

School-aged children are confronted with new and widening opportunities as their world begins to blossom. School cafeterias, slumber party invitations, field trips, and bus rides enter your child's world. While exciting, these new situations are often frightening for parents of food-allergic children. Parents who found raising a preschooler challenging suddenly realize that there was at least some peace during that time, as they alone controlled the child's environment. Now, parents are confronted with new environments and social norms that require constant risk assessment and management. Your child's own wishes and desires also need to be considered during this time. Suddenly, life can become very complicated and frightening.

During this stage, for your child's well-being and continued normal development, he or she should be encouraged to take an increasingly major role in his or her own care. A child needs to continue taking age-appropriate control of his or her own food allergies. This will involve communicating needs to others, reading food labels, and eventually being responsible for carrying the EpiPen and learning how to self-administer the injection if possible or absolutely necessary. Many parents are asked by caregivers at what age a child should be expected to assess a reaction, make a decision, and actually administer the EpiPen. It is unwise for caregivers to ask this in an effort to pass on this responsibility to the child and free themselves from this aspect of care. Doctors do not usually give a definite age as to when it might be appropriate to self-administer the EpiPen, as individual maturity varies greatly. Although it is wise for your child to know how to use the EpiPen if absolutely necessary, it is not generally safe to allow a child to make the decision whether to administer a painful injection during a physical crisis. The question also becomes irrelevant as a child or an adult can experience loss of consciousness as a symptom of anaphylaxis.

A conflict can arise when parents attempt to manage the child's allergies in the same ways they did when the child was three years old. Your job should still include making the safest possible environment for your child to grow and thrive in, but different methods may be called for. Your work may be more concentrated at the school level, communicating with other children's parents and with sports coaches rather than physically supervising your child at every moment. This "letting go" process can be torturous, but what is the alternative?

Providing 100 percent safety is not possible, because some measure of risk is present in every situation, even when you're with your child. A previously safe food may be contaminated at the manufacturing level, or you might sometimes forget to bring the EpiPen with you. We are human. We can strive to have our children "safe enough." If you don't have some sense of safety about a given situation, perhaps your child should not participate, or your presence is necessary. Many parents opt for home schooling after an attempt to create a safe enough environment at school is not successful. Others weigh their child's unique needs and the level of cooperation they received from the school and ultimately feel that their child is indeed safe enough.

Living with "safe enough" is extremely stressful. We as parents often second-guess our risk assessments and decisions at every turn. In the early years through kindergarten, take advantage of other young children's natural acceptance of food allergies in your child. Many parents report that young friends who have been educated about food allergies quickly become your child's best allies in avoiding exposure. These friends have even been known to remind their adult parents of the need to safely include your child in various activities.

Unfortunately, this acceptance sometimes gives way to teasing, bullying, and making your child feel different, beginning around fourth grade and escalating until around seventh grade, when it can drop off considerably. Your child, who may have always accepted and managed his or her allergy remarkably well, might respond by becoming angry about having to cope with his or her food allergy. This is normal and should be supported.

Of course, any child would rather not have to deal with limitations and feeling different from others. Validate and support your child's feelings. Sympathize with the wish to eliminate the allergy, but be careful not to instill any false hope. Providing your child with individual or group counseling, as well as participating in a support group, may be helpful. Encourage your child to be involved with people who support and accept him or her unconditionally, and in time your child will come to accept the food allergy again.

AGE ELEVEN AND UP

Adolescence may mean a time of less parental management of allergies as the growing child begins to take full responsibility for preventing reactions and surrounds him- or herself with others who can help recognize and treat an allergic reaction. Yet, the normal developmental elements that accompany adolescence might also be working against this transition. Adolescence is a time of struggle between independence and dependence, when peer relationships and social interaction become central in your child's life and the likelihood of experimentation increases.

Food allergies may heighten the age-old struggle between autonomy and dependence. Just when children may need more space and control in their lives, their food allergies are a source of worry and concern, keeping them close to their parents. This may be felt by both parents and adolescents. It is difficult to grant the appropriate increase in freedom when there is a simultaneous increase in risk.

Suddenly, there are new risks to consider. Will your adolescent or those around him or her be tempted to consume alcohol? Alcohol and drugs could cause the adolescent to become impaired, clouding his or her judgment. An error in judgment could lead to an accidental exposure to an offending food or an inability to recognize and treat a reaction. Even kissing has been reported to cause serious allergic reactions if the adolescent's partner has consumed an offending food.

Adolescents may begin to question what they have been told about their food allergies. This questioning may lead the adolescent to reject his or her food allergies. This is similar to the way in which some diabetic adolescents have been known to reject the diabetes by disregarding food restrictions, not properly monitoring their blood sugar level, and skipping insulin injections. Adolescents with food allergies could virtually hold their parents hostage by disregarding dietary restrictions or refusing to carry their EpiPen.

How your child's friends perceive food allergies will greatly affect his or her own acceptance of the allergies. Adolescents feel the need to "fit in," and having food allergies may make this difficult. Many parents report that the increase in social activity is problematic because many of these activities seem to include or revolve around food.

Again, open and honest communication will aid in the transition into adolescence. Many parents feel that clear communication beginning early in the child's life made adolescence easier to live through for everyone involved.

Allowing age-appropriate control of food allergies throughout childhood will minimize the difficulties experienced in adolescence. Acceptance by the adolescent as well as acceptance by friends and family also help adolescence go more smoothly. For parents, surviving your food-allergic child's adolescence requires guts and prayers. It is bound to be difficult to give up control of the allergy management to your adolescent even if you have prepared for this since the day of the initial diagnosis. Receiving support while your adolescent achieves independence is vital, as it is for any parent of a non–food-allergic child.

TRUST

One developmental factor that has not yet been discussed and that plays an essential role through all the stages of development is establishing trust early on and maintaining it into adulthood. There are enormous implications for the food-allergic child if this trust is not gained and held. Having trust in others conveys that the world is a trustworthy place to explore on his or her own. Trust is crucial to the process of developing autonomy. Trust is also a necessary element in developing hope, a core ego strength. In *The Life Cycle Completed,* E. H. Erikson writes, "Hope is the expectation that . . . good things will happen in the future. Hope enables the child to move forward into the world and take up new challenges."

In managing food allergies, there are ample risks to establishing and maintaining trust at every stage of development and in every situation the child encounters. Consider the necessary elements in developing trust.

Starting in the first year, a child's sense of trust is becoming established in his or her growing faith in the stability of the world. Erikson explains that this begins with interactions between the parents and child. He writes that the child must learn that the parents are dependable and therefore trustworthy. This dependability, he believes, comes from the parents behaving consistently and predictably relieving any discomfort felt by the child.

A child who has suffered an anaphylactic reaction early on may come away from the experience feeling that caregivers are not always dependable or predictable. Subsequently, parents who teach their children to be extremely cautious are, through their words and attitude, confirming the child's observation that caregivers may not be dependable and predictable. This pattern suggesting that the world may not be a safe place is a direct barrier to developing trust.

My own son experienced a trust-breaking experience at age four, when a well-intentioned preschool teacher became alarmed when she thought there may have been an offending ingredient in a cookie she had given him. Max needed to spit it out quickly and be carried to the nearest bathroom, where she washed his mouth out. The teacher then watched nervously for any reaction. Max was understandably surprised, embarrassed, and scared. He did not know if he was about to finally experience getting the shot we had discussed and be whisked away in an ambulance to the hospital or not. Fortunately, there was no reaction. The label read "may contain peanuts," though evidently there were no peanuts present. If there had been, even the act of washing his mouth out would not have prevented a reaction.

At first I was upset that the incident had occurred, but accidents happen, and I was pleased that the teacher had been concerned and had quickly taken action. After joining my son in his feeling of having been let down, I mentioned that the teacher's caring enough about him to take quick action was a reason to trust her. He still expressed feelings of being angry and seemed to lose some trust in that teacher as a result of the experience.

After that, I saw the teacher actively trying to reestablish trust. However, I have also seen my son grow more wary of trusting others and nervous about being surprised in that way again. In one way I am glad to see him being so careful, but in another I feel sad that he struggles with trust and will most likely encounter this type of situation again.

Ultimately, trust depends on your own sense that what you are doing is right. This can be difficult, however, in a society with little understanding of anaphylaxis. There will always be people, even other parents of food-allergic children, who challenge and criticize the decisions a parent makes. For example, if you decide not to send your food-allergic child to preschool, you may be criticized for coddling or sheltering your child too much. If you decide to send him or her to preschool, you might be chastised for putting your child at risk.

This constant second-guessing and barrage of conflicting and unsupported comments from extended family members, friends, neighbors, school systems, and even physicians leave many parents feeling battered and bruised. Being in this position may also eat away at parents' confidence and have an effect on the child's sense of trust in his or her parents and the world. Complicating this dilemma is the heightened need for a high level of trust in all caregivers that a child at risk for experiencing an anaphylactic reaction requires.

Developing trust in themselves is also crucial for normal child development from birth to adolescence. Children at risk for experiencing anaphylaxis need to trust in their own judgment as to which people are worthy of their trust. Each day a food-allergic child needs to reevaluate this decision to trust that the food that a person is giving him or her is safe. After many successful interactions with the same person, a child may begin to feel more comfortable with the decision to trust that person.

THE SILVER LINING

Despite the challenges, there can be positive aspects to dealing with severe food allergies. Children who cope successfully with food allergies from an early age often have a level of maturity and sensitivity far beyond their chronological age. Because of the self-discipline required in addition to the normal challenges of growing up, food-allergic children often become stronger, more self-assured people. The ongoing need for communication between themselves and others contributes to their ability to relate well to other people. The need to communicate among family members can provide a satisfying sense of cohesion and belonging.

Food-allergic children also need to identify and cultivate

"real" friends. By learning what to look for in others—qualities like cooperation, accommodation, and compassion—food-allergic children in turn have these same qualities to offer. The same goes for parents. We have the opportunity to make deep and rewarding connections with the many people who go above and beyond the call of duty for our children. Few if any parents would not trade their child's food allergies for the chance to give their child a "normal" carefree childhood. But the resulting positive impact on their precious child's character would not be traded for anything.

5

BRANCHING OUT— WORKING WITH CAREGIVERS AND SCHOOLS

————— ∿ —————

AT SOME POINT, you may want or need to make arrangements to have another adult be responsible for your child in your absence. This other adult might be a baby-sitter, a family member, a day care professional, or a teacher. Ideally, this alternative caregiver will have accurate knowledge about food allergies, anaphylaxis, food avoidance management, symptom recognition, and reaction treatment. Realistically, this is often not the case. Until there is a greater general knowledge about food allergies, the responsibility for educating others falls on individual families.

TO LEAVE OR NOT TO LEAVE

Parents report feeling very differently about the possibility of arranging child care for their food-allergic children. Some assess their child's unique concerns and avoid leaving their child in another's care until absolutely necessary. Other parents' assessments lead them to continue arranging child care just as they would for a nonallergic child. Whatever your position on the matter, consider your own well-being in the decision because your well-being has a direct effect on your child's level of safety and happiness.

If you feel you must supervise your child at all times, be sure to recognize when you need a break and find the resources to arrange one for yourself. If you feel your child needs to participate in a child care arrangement but the stress and worry you feel reaches an intolerable level, listen to your fears. You may need to change the situation in order to meet your standards for safety. When the stress level is tolerable, your child is probably in a "safe enough" situation.

The first step in arranging alternative care is to educate yourself. Know exactly what you are dealing with before you communicate your child's needs to others. This means learning about food allergies and anaphylaxis and understanding the process you and your family are going through and the role you play in managing your child's food allergies. In educating yourself, you may find that what you need from a caregiver becomes remarkably clear. By having a full understanding yourself, you may feel empowered and able to see that your child's needs are met.

To establish what type of care is feasible for your child, assess your child's unique allergies and other factors such as age, number and severity of allergies, what you are comfortable with, and your budget. It may be that your child has multiple severe allergies and is only one year old. In this case you may be comfortable leaving your child only with a close relative in your home. Another parent in the same circumstances may need to go to work full-time and, because of financial constraints, must consider a day care center. Still another parent may choose to consider a small licensed day care provider in the caregiver's home.

Choose the appropriate child care situation for you and your child first and then investigate the people involved in your choices. Although there seem to be risks inherent in situations where a larger number of children are cared for outside of the home, in the end, the capabilities of the person in charge of the situation and your child are the best indicator of risk.

The caregiver's willing attitude and competence are the keys to providing safety for your child. It is helpful if the person has previous knowledge about food allergies, but only if it is complete and accurate knowledge that leads to the implementation of appropriate safety measures. A person previously unaware of food allergies may be just as competent, if not more competent, in managing food allergies, once he or she is educated.

It is important to find a willing and cooperative caregiver, but this willingness must be accompanied by the ability to take in the information and follow through with risk assessment and risk management. That person must understand how the information about food allergies affects the care of the child and find ways to keep the child safe. Many parents are so elated when a potential caregiver seems open and confident about managing food allergies that they stop their assessment of the person there. Look for signs that the caregiver has incorporated food allergy education into the care of your child. For example, seemingly wonderful caregivers may incorrectly instruct you to leave your EpiPen at home, thinking they will call you if they need it; or they may think it is enough not to give your child an offending food, but then allow toddlers who have full run of the area to snack on foods containing offending ingredients. Cooperation should not be confused with competent cooperation.

EDUCATE THE CAREGIVER

It is important to educate the chosen caregiver with information about food allergies and anaphylaxis in general as well as your child's specialized concerns. Provide the caregiver with information available from the Food Allergy Network. Specifically, the Day Care and Preschool Guide to Managing Food Allergies is a must for any caregiver. Share this information with a potential caregiver even if it is your own mother or teenage baby-sitter. It is useful to provide this information to a caregiver before a scheduled meeting to allow for "digestion" of the material. This will also weed out any caregivers who may not be fit to provide necessary care and allow those who are capable to form some educated questions for you.

Arrange a meeting between you and the potential caregiver to discuss the specifics of your child's needs, including all offending ingredients and severity of allergies. Share everything you have learned about methods of safely managing food avoidance. Together with the caregiver, come up with guidelines for how food will be dealt with. Make a risk assessment of the environment and the routine, identifying potential risks to your child. Consider who will provide food, crafts, and activities that may involve offending ingredients or cross-contamination from counters, tables, and other children. Discuss holiday and birthday celebrations, substitute caregivers, and field trips, if applicable. Create guidelines to minimize existing risks.

The discussion should also include possible allergic reaction symptoms, assessment of symptoms, and emergency procedures. Create a clear emergency procedure flyer that is posted in a conspicuous place. The Food Allergy Network has an efficient "Emergency Health Care Plan" available, which is a form you can fill out based on your child's specific needs. The form identifies trained staff members and lists exactly what your child is allergic to, the possible symptoms of an allergic reaction, what action should be taken, such as medications to be administered and calling the rescue squad, and emergency contacts, complete with phone numbers. This form is complete on one page with your child's picture at the top and should be signed by you as well as your child's allergist. Your child's allergist needs to have some sort of contact with the caregiver, even if it is only his or her signature on the emergency flyer. This signature validates that there is a genuine medical threat to your child and establishes the need for lifesaving action to be taken. Ideally, a doctor or nurse would instruct the caregiver in the proper procedure for administering the EpiPen. Realistically, this may have to be done by you. The use of a video and obtaining a "trainer" EpiPen that operates just like a real EpiPen but does not contain medication or a needle can enhance your demonstration. Impress upon the caregiver the importance of administering the EpiPen injection as soon as a serious reaction is recognized. Also, let the caregiver know that it is better to administer epinephrine unnecessarily, as no harm will come to the child, than to err in not administering the EpiPen when it might be necessary.

In the case of a licensed day care provider with a certified assistant or a day care center where several people may provide care for your child, arrangements need to be made to convey this necessary information to all of those people as well.

Your Role

Your role in dealing with the potential caregiver is to educate, clearly state what your child will require, and offer support in the form of information and understanding. Not everyone is cut out to properly care for a child with severe food allergies. When you feel you have found someone who is, think of that person as your partner in keeping your child safe and happy.

After discussing the pertinent information, ask the caregiver if he or she feels confident about providing the necessary care for your child. This includes your own family members! Offer appreciation for the caregiver's willingness to take on the additional responsibility. Always be available to answer any questions that come up. The caregiver may need more support at the start of providing care when questions may arise. Most caregivers will feel more comfortable and confident with the arrangement over time.

Monitor and Evaluate

Monitor and evaluate the care your child is receiving. Look for specific ways in which your caregiver has reduced the risk to your child. Be sure that the caregiver's actions are consistent with what they claim to know about food allergies. Make sure you get the distinct feeling that the caregiver "gets it."

If you do not feel more confident and comfortable over time, this may be a sign that this is not the best situation at this time and other arrangements might need to be considered. Arranging care is stressful and demands an enormous amount of your time and energy, but do not be afraid to start over.

Potential problems with alternative caregivers may range from an unwillingness to care for your child or a refusal to take responsibility for administering the EpiPen to disbelief regarding your information about food allergies. Some providers have asked parents to sign a legal waiver releasing the caregiver from any liability for failing to properly administer emergency treatment.

Many parents report facing varying degrees of resistance when attempting to arrange child care. Some resistance is subtle, as when the caregiver is willing to provide care but will not commit to carrying through with any necessary safety measures. Some resistance is blatant, as in the case of a New York kindergartner who was refused admittance to a private kindergarten solely because of his food allergies.

Legal Questions

Legal questions involving laypeople administering the lifesaving EpiPen are also common. Legal waivers waiving your right to ever take any legal action are sometimes asked for. The basic rule of thumb is that parents should not agree to sign any release of liability. Other legal questions tend to be complicated, as many feel that the laws relevant to children with "disabilities" are ambiguous, with the very definition of *disability* open to interpretation. Understandably, some parents may be reluctant to label their food-allergic child as having a disability, but in this way they may be entitled to protection from discrimination if a day care center or school refuses them entry or refuses to make necessary adaptations for them by providing them with a safe place to eat or being willing to keep and administer the EpiPen. Some advocates and parents feel that food allergies should be considered a disability in the eyes of the law in order to ensure that the children's risks are addressed and to offer them protection from discrimination. They feel that these children should be protected under Section 504 of the Rehabilitation Act of 1973, as a disability is defined as a physical impairment that severely limits one or more major life activities such as breathing, eating, and going to school. Not everyone agrees with this interpretation, as the courts have sometimes ruled that food allergies do not meet the definition of a disability, stating that allergies limit the major life activities only "a little bit," but not severely. The legal wranglings are sure to continue, and hopefully more rights and protection will ultimately be provided specifically for children with food allergies. In the interim, you may want to look to Section 504 mentioned above, as well as the Americans with Disabilities Act of 1990, as they do provide guidelines for care.

Legal questions aside, only you can decide if it is in your child's best interest to pursue any given battle that you may encounter. Your child's immediate need for a safe and welcoming environment supersedes any legal concerns. Yet, those few who choose to fight may be the ones who succeed in providing more rights and protection for all of our children with food allergies. The legal picture of food allergies is a dynamic one, and for current information or if you have a specific question you may want to contact the Food Allergy Network for resources in your area. You can also receive additional information by contacting educational rights specialist Ellie Goldberg, M.Ed., of Healthy Kids: The Key to Basics, listed in the resource section of this book.

Convincing Others

Difficulty in convincing others of the potential seriousness of food allergies is the most common problem experienced by parents. This may be one of the most stressful and frustrating components associated with managing food allergies. In an ideal world, every individual would be aware of the dangers associated with food allergies. Until that level of awareness occurs, it is up to us to face the ignorance, which feels like resistance.

Many people have their own ideas about what allergies are all about. They may base their knowledge on a limited experience of their own or one other person's experience of allergies. Many times this does not include the risk for a serious and fatal reaction. People often do not realize how even a tiny amount of food can cause a reaction. We are often accused of being "crazy," hysterical, and overprotective.

A vicious cycle may result when parents get stuck in the same ineffective response to resistance. The other person may make the parents feel as if they are acting "crazy" or overreacting. As parents are angered or frustrated that they are not getting their concerns across, they may feel the need to "increase the volume" and make more demands in a way that is perceived by the other person to be even more hysterical. If the other person is not understanding the reality of the situation and is faced with parents who he or she feels are acting crazy, the person is more apt to dismiss or reject what the parents are saying. Then the parents are perplexed as to why, after being even more deliberate in voicing their concerns, the person appears to be even less concerned. Now the communication is stuck in an unproductive place, and any hope of establishing communication is diminished.

If you are faced with this situation, be calm. De-escalate the tension by using statements such as, "You'd think that was the case; unfortunately, there may be other considerations." Find an impartial way of creating a context to share general knowledge about the seriousness of food allergies. Ask the person if he or she would mind spending a few minutes on something that could be very important to your child. Then you could share pertinent videos or written materials that the person could look at alone before the next contact.

Once you have made available a formal, unbiased resource, try to have another discussion where you may add the specifics of your own child's allergies. You may be surprised that the person is more open and full of questions. If not, this person may be too rigid in his or her beliefs to integrate the newly received information. Exclude him or her from providing care for your child. Either way, you will be moving closer to making the right decision for your child's care.

WORKING WITH SCHOOLS

Schools are notorious for causing undue frustrations and risks for the families of food-allergic children. Perhaps you already have one or more horror stories to share. In general, schools and other institutions are seldom well informed or supportive about methods of ensuring safety for a child with food allergies. This is changing as our numbers grow and schools are forced to become educated and make provisions to safely include food-allergic students.

It seems as if schools have recently been asked to do more with less and less. Schools may feel burdened by being asked to handle other children with special needs such as attention deficit disorder. Plus, they're managing before- and after-school programs with fewer resources than ever before. Having a school nurse and staff available to create and implement a safety plan for the child might seem like a luxury that the school cannot afford. These are just some of the factors that make most schools unnecessarily risky for children with severe food allergies.

In a study of fatal and near-fatal anaphylactic reactions published in 1992, noted earlier in this book, four of six children who died experienced the fatal anaphylactic reaction at school. This fact, coupled with the fact that none of the seven near-fatal reactions occurred at school, raises a question about the ability of school health care systems to deal with such medical emergencies.

You might think that having a parent nearby during a reaction would increase the odds for survival. However, at least one parent was present during three of the six children's fatal reactions and four of the seven children's near-fatal reactions. It is more likely that the factor linked to survivability was the location of the reactions. The reactions occurring at private residences were more likely to be quickly recognized, assessed, and treated as medical emergencies.

In the public setting of school, the amount of time necessary to recognize and treat the symptoms was clearly compromised. None of the children who died received an EpiPen injection before severe respiratory symptoms developed, whereas all the children who experienced near-fatal reactions received an EpiPen before or within five minutes of the onset of severe respiratory symptoms.

The potentially lifesaving action of administering an EpiPen in a timely manner, particularly while a child is at school, seems to have many barriers. One barrier is the general lack of awareness of the potential seriousness of food allergies. In most cases, it is up to you to educate your child's school about food allergies.

To Ban or Not to Ban?

For many cities and towns, preschools and elementary schools, that is the question. There exists a fierce and sometimes mean-spirited debate about banning certain food items in some communities. Begun by parents who long for safety, along with well-intentioned administrators, all hell has broken loose in some communities, where restrictions are placed on unaware and misinformed parents. The debate is often fueled by the media's love of controversy. They quickly pick up on a story about an innocuous food item loaded with warm childhood memories, and the power of the state, in a situation where the lives of children are at stake. Their reports pit parents against parents.

Bans on peanuts and peanut butter are the most common, as these are the most common allergens as well as the most lethal. At first glance, the ban might seem like the solution that parents of allergic children are looking for, but many parents find themselves unwittingly placed in the middle of a brawl that is counterproductive to their desire to provide safety and acceptance for their child. Parents advocating a ban may be faced with hostile parents who resent the fact that their children's freedom is being restricted. These parents are then less likely to be open to education and cooperation. Nobody likes to be told what to do, especially when it comes to their children. Many times a ban on certain foods is presented in such a heavy-handed way to the overwhelming majority of parents of nonallergic children that outrage and misunderstanding are the usual reactions. Most of those parents may not be educated about the dangers that these foods pose to food-allergic children and simply do not understand the grave risk to this relatively small number of children. Many believe their children have the right to eat whatever they wish, proclaiming that peanut butter is the only lunch item that their children will eat and that the smaller number of children with food allergies should make the necessary sacrifices, such as not attending school or not eating in the cafeteria.

Another reason why a peanut ban may not provide the necessary level of safety is the risk that some administrators will use the ban as a substitute for a systemwide safety protocol. There might be a tendency to see the ban as a simple solution, without any education for the staff and students, without any plans to enforce the ban or contingency plans for when banned items are brought in, and without any safety protocols or emergency plans in case of a reaction. If you are a parent of a food-allergic child who attends school in an allergy-ban environment, whether it is only in the classroom or schoolwide, be sure that all the other bases have been covered, as there is the danger of a false sense of security for you, the child, and the staff, even when intentions are good. A ban should not be a replacement for safety protocols, as accidental ingestion or exposure is never planned or intended.

The next reason for not encouraging a ban concerns the issue of how far the bans should go. If a ban is implemented for peanut allergies, what about the next child to come along, like mine, who also has an allergy to tree nuts? And what about the child who is allergic to milk, eggs, or soy? If each item is banned, what will the majority of children be able to eat while at school?

Possibly the best reason that the ban may not provide the greatest degree of safety is the logistical improbability of actually providing a safe environment. Even in the most favorable of situations, where parents are educated and willing to be empathetic and cooperative, and where the decision to ban peanuts is made in collaboration with other parents, it still may not work, or it may have so many gaps in safety that it might not be worth it. As many parents of food-allergic children can attest, providing an allergy-free environment even in your own home is an almost impossible task, even when you practice extreme vigilance. We are many times supereducated, drawing on years of education as to what may or may not be safe, dealing with ever-changing labels, cross-contamination problems in our own kitchens, and allergens showing up in surprising places every day. How can we reasonably expect this same kind of knowledge and effort from the parents of nonallergic children? Even in my own extended family, coordinating a peanut- and tree-nut-free holiday has proven difficult at best and impossible at worst.

Imagine planning one safe holiday dinner with extended family as a microcosm of what you could expect on a daily basis at school. Think about what it is like to coordinate a safe meal prepared by many people. There are usually countless questions, unread labels that defy suspicion, risks for cross-contamination in food preparation, and misinformation due to rapid changes in food production facts. This could play out with family members innocently not checking the label of jelly beans, since one would never dream that jelly beans could contain peanut oil. A brownie mix that you had previously communicated was safe may turn up reading "may contain nuts" on the label this week. There could be cross-contamination on kitchen bowls and utensils when a relative makes a special nut-free batch of cookies, if it is prepared immediately following a batch that did contain nuts. Well-meaning family members may inadvertently put your child at risk for reaction. And then there is almost always a distant uncle or aunt who cannot, or will not, believe the seriousness of the allergy and feels that having mixed nuts or chestnuts on Thanksgiving is a tradition that he or she is unwilling to forgo. In any population, there are bound to be those people who will go out of their way to try to be helpful, and those who may go out of their way not to be helpful, and everything in between. You can expect this at the school level as well. The fact is that even if the entire population had good intentions, it would not necessarily keep children safe.

If your food-allergic child attends a school with a ban in place in addition to having all the education and safety protocols in place, good for you! It is not impossible for a ban to be presented in the correct way, be well supported by cooperation and enforcement, and to have contingency and emergency protocols in place. It is simply not likely for the average school system to provide this. You are in the extraordinary and enviable minority. However, watch for signs of trouble in the child who is growing older and may begin to resent the attention that comes from being the cause of the ban. There is a point where the physical benefits may not be worth the emotional price for the older child. By this time they may very well be more ready to manage food avoidance on their own in conjunction with other safety protocols.

STRIVING FOR SAFETY: AN ALTERNATIVE TO A BAN

Adaptations in the classroom and schools should be requested and granted, but a ban may not be the answer if your goal is to increase safety through education and cooperation without singling out your child any more than is necessary. Instead of asking for a ban, it might be more effective to ask for a minimizing of the offending food item. Every effort to minimize will greatly reduce the risk to your child.

There is no one solution for every child and every school. Assess your child's unique needs based on age, the severity of past reactions, and the likelihood of sensitivity to the mere touch or smell of allergens. The environment should also be assessed as to the size of the population, the resources available to it, and the anticipated level of cooperation from parents and staff. Only then should a combination of approaches and adaptations available to the system be decided upon. For instance, different solutions are called for when contrasting the needs of a touch- and smell-sensitive preschooler in a small environment of one teacher, one room, and six other students, versus a fifth-grader in a large elementary school that provides lunch to hundreds of students and a staff of over a hundred people. All kinds of provisions can be made. However, every solution should involve certain precautions, the education of all staff, and a concrete emergency plan put in place. The goal should be to minimize the possibility of an accidental reaction, but to be completely prepared to recognize, treat, and act on an emergency plan if a reaction should arise.

The most efficient way to reduce risk to peanut-allergic students is for the school itself to make the decision to not offer the obvious peanut products for snack or lunch items. There are usually so many other alternatives in a cafeteria that they would be missed only until a child has a new favorite. This is different from a ban in that students are not prohibited from bringing those products in from home, but it greatly minimizes the risk to the allergic student. It also succeeds in sending a message to every other student and parent. It says, we understand the risks and this is our way of helping to minimize the risks to this child, without placing harsh restrictions on the majority of the students. However, obtaining this type of provision is more easily said than done, as there still appears to be great resistance to the elimination of that all-time favorite, peanut butter, even in the face of grave risk to our youngsters.

Parents must consider every aspect of school life, from snack and lunch protocols to art supply ingredients and learning aids. There are so many considerations and adaptations that it is not feasible to cover them all here. The Food Allergy Network's School Food Allergy Program and the Day Care and Preschool Guide to Managing Food Allergies are probably the two best resources available.

At my son's school a number of provisions have evolved over the last three years. (Keep in mind that he is in the second grade.) We are fortunate to have a full-time nurse present at school. My son's school nurse has been extremely compassionate and willing to learn about food allergies and go forward with new policies to improve safety. One of the adaptations we have made is the creation of a peanut-free table in the cafeteria, where my son is joined by friends who do not have any peanut- or tree-nut-containing foods in their lunches. Although there are other lunch periods before and after my son's scheduled lunch time, peanut and tree-nut products are never allowed at this designated table to help eliminate the possibility of peanut residue on the table itself. The janitorial staff is aware of the situation and keeps this table especially clean. All teachers and staff have been educated about food allergies by the school nurse and have taken the initiative in checking food items of the children who wish to sit at this particular table.

All staff know how to recognize Max and a possible reaction if they saw him having any symptoms at recess, art, music, gym, or in the boys' restroom. By law in Massachusetts, the school nurse is able to train and delegate other teachers to administer the EpiPen if necessary. The children in Max's class have been educated about food allergies each year, and a letter is sent home to parents making them aware of this health risk. In this letter they are invited to do their part in helping keep my son's classroom as safe as possible. There is an EpiPen and liquid antihistamine in his classroom as well as in the nurse's office. An emergency procedure flyer, complete with all of my son's important information and phone numbers, as well as his picture, is posted in the school office, the nurse's office, and the classroom.

My son does not eat anything brought in by another student unless there is written permission from me indicating that I have spoken to the parents and feel it will indeed be safe. There is a container that I have sent in with safe snacks for him to tap into when food items that may be unsafe are sent in. Snacks are brought in from home and parents and children are encouraged to save any unsafe snacks for the cafeteria. But when unsafe snacks do make their way into the classroom, there is a standardized way of dealing with it: that student is sent to a back table where he or she will eat his or her snack and wash the table as well as his or her hands when finished. It is agreed that I will chaperone all field trips as an extra precaution when the children are away from school and the school nurse. Max's teachers have been very willing to become educated about food allergies and become responsible caregivers. Each year there is a reeducation process and negotiation with the new teacher as to what protocols he or she is willing to have in place. These protocols are based on past success and are arrived at in cooperation with the teacher, the nurse, and myself, keeping the individual teacher's preferences in mind.

The following is an example of an important letter that this year's teacher sent home to parents in order to raise awareness and invite cooperation. Originally written by Max's kindergarten teacher, Ms. Lawless, it has been edited each year.

Dear Parent(s),

I would like to make you aware of a health issue that the children are learning about this year. One of our classmates, Max Collins, has a severe food allergy to peanuts and tree nuts, their products, and oils. Strict avoidance is the only way to prevent an allergic reaction. The allergy is life threatening. For this reason we must be most cautious with the classroom snacks and party foods. Snacks are eaten here in our classroom daily. Your child is still welcome to bring peanut snack items from home. However, each time he or she chooses to bring a snack without peanuts or nuts, your child plays an important part in decreasing the risk to Max. When a child celebrates a birthday, it is a common practice for parents to send cupcakes or special snacks. Parents are welcome to continue this practice. Due to the risk of cross-contamination from the kitchen counters and utensils, and the fact that peanuts turn up in the most unlikely places, such as plain M&M's, Max may often eat his own safe alternative treat.

Max's mom, Lisa Collins, will be the room mother this year and will be contacting parents to provide treats for the holiday parties. Mrs. Collins can provide you with information regarding safe brands of foods. She invites you to call her at xxx-xxxx with any questions or concerns. We want Max to participate fully in all of our class activities this year. With your help, we can keep our classroom safe for everyone.

I am most appreciative of your understanding and cooperation.

Your Child's Teacher

I know of many situations where schools may go to even greater lengths to provide safety to food-allergic children and still others that have done much less. It is up to you to work with what you are presented, working with the school to continue to make improvements each year. Living with some anxiety is a given, and a parent can always think of further provisions that could be made. We must struggle to find the balance between trying to make the child's environment as safe as possible without pushing too hard and losing the cooperation we need.

GETTING HELP

The American Academy of Pediatrics and the American Academy of Allergy, Asthma, and Immunology have issued position statements for the treatment of anaphylaxis in the schools. Included in the American Academy of Pediatrics guidelines is the recommendation that an anaphylaxis kit be kept in each school and that the kits be made available to a school nurse and/or two trained staff members. The guidelines also recommend that two staff member volunteers be trained in an emergency care program and that anaphylaxis recognition and treatment be included in that program. The problem is that few school officials know these guidelines exist.

As a result of the low level of awareness of anaphylaxis and the guidelines available to them, many schools are reluctant to accommodate children with this "hidden" disability. Another reason for the reluctance seems to be the schools' fear of liability if they are involved in administering the EpiPen.

Many parents of food-allergic children have found that schools are reluctant to assume the responsibility to administer the potentially lifesaving EpiPen. The absence of a full-time nurse in many schools across the country may be one contributing factor. School nurses should refer to their State Nurse Practice Act and Medical Practice Acts for guidance in the administration of medication. If the Nurse Practice Act prohibits the nurse from delegating and training other staff members in the administering of an EpiPen, then the school must meet its obligation to students, as required by federal law, by hiring a person who is licensed to administer the medication.

Sometimes, lay staff members think they cannot legally administer any medication, and they fear being liable if they would take action. This is usually not the case. At the very least, many states offer lay staff members protection from liability in the form of a "Good Samaritan Act."

I experienced a tense situation when I refused to sign a medical waiver at my son's prospective preschool. The preschool was attempting to cover their own liability in the worst-case scenario. I received the advice that I could not release the school from providing necessary medical care for my child. This situation was eventually resolved, but it was not the way I had envisioned my son beginning preschool.

One mother shared with me her story of how her kindergarten-aged daughter cried incessantly when she dropped her off at school. This crying persisted over a long period of time. It turned out that the school was refusing to keep the child's EpiPen on site. She had every right to cry, as she did not feel safe.

Choose Your Battles

Painful and *frustrating* are two words parents use to describe the experience of dealing with resistance so often, about a matter of such vital concern. If people refuse to accept the realities of food allergies, it is as if they are rejecting part of what makes up your child as an individual. Divorcing yourself from the emotions involved in order to go forward is difficult and potentially harmful.

It is up to you to decide when and how to manage resistance. Even if every law is on your side, it is up to you to decide whether a situation is worth fighting for. Fighting back is one tactic that may ultimately improve the quality of life for other food-allergic children coming up, but do not feel as though you must fight every resistance. Knowing how to choose your battles helps to ensure that some sort of balance and peace is experienced in the entire family. Remember the powerful tactic of sharing your knowledge and expressing your disappointment when a person has not considered the best interest of your child after becoming educated.

If you are facing resistance from school officials or other caregivers—or if you simply want them to know more about food allergies—I invite you to recommend that they read this book, particularly the next chapter. As the next chapter, for caregivers, is the final one, this will be my last opportunity to convey my thoughts directly to you, the parent of a food-allergic child. I wish to extend my heartfelt empathy for the challenges you now face and the ones you will face in the future. If I could leave you with one thought it would be to treasure and value your child. Although one can write an entire book about food allergies, it is but one small part of what makes your child unique. Create a safe environment so that you and your child can get on with the business of discovering and enjoying all the other wonderful qualities that make your child who he or she is. Recognize and value all these parts and soon your child, and everyone around him or her, will do the same.

6

FOR
CAREGIVERS

———— ∾ ————

PERHAPS YOU ALREADY KNOW about food allergies and the impact they have on the care you provide for a food-allergic child. Or perhaps you're learning for the first time that an otherwise harmless ingredient can put a child's life in jeopardy. Either way, you may have lots of questions.

When Patricia Schaffer, director of a Kinder Care Learning Center in Littleton, Colorado, was asked what she believed to be most important to share with other caregivers, she answered, "Take it [food allergy] seriously and know what to do. You *can* deal with it. It's not something you can ignore."

The care, as well as the quality of care you provide, is vital to the food-allergic child and his or her family. Keep in mind that the information contained here is not intended to be a substitute for information provided by the food-allergic child's physician. All matters of health require medical supervision.

If you haven't done so, please review carefully the basic food allergy information presented in chapter 1. This will empower you to communicate better with the parents of a food-allergic child as well as to aid you in making the best possible decisions for practical daily living. While this guide is not a comprehensive resource on the medical management of food allergies, there are a number of safety tips to follow when caring for a child with severe food allergies.

Managing Food Avoidance

The first important step in caring for a food-allergic child is learning and practicing food avoidance. After you acquire full and accurate information regarding food allergies and understand the needs of the child's family, it is time to do some serious work. Think about every aspect of the care you provide and look for any potential gaps in safety.

Increases in Risk

Factors that could increase risk include:

⬥ The presence of any other individual during the care

⬥ Any variation in the normal routine, such as a field trip

⬥ Any occasion when food is provided by anyone other than the affected child's parents.

⬥ Any time offending ingredients are present on site, regardless of whether the child is present, as there is a risk of cross-contamination on surfaces, clothes, and other individuals' bodies

⬥ Any circumstances that might hinder your ability to avoid offending foods, recognize the symptoms of a reaction, administer prompt treatment, or transport the child to an emergency room

✧ Any obstacles to necessary and frequent communication between parent and caregiver

TO DECREASE POTENTIAL RISKS

Below are some ways to decrease the risk of an allergic reaction to a child in your care. A comprehensive guide that is a must for any caregiver is *The Daycare and Preschool Guide to Managing Food Allergies,* available from the Food Allergy Network. To decrease potential risks:

✧ Become educated about food allergies and anaphylaxis.

✧ Become aware of every form that an offending ingredient can take and learn what words to look for on ingredient labels.

✧ Arrange a meeting with parents to discuss the specifics of the child's history of allergies and brainstorm methods of providing safety with the parents.

✧ Educate any and all caregivers, adults, and children and even parents of other children present. A great resource for educating children is a video available from the Food Allergy Network entitled "Alexander, the Elephant Who Couldn't Eat Peanuts." Companion children's books and a teaching guide are also available.

✧ Create a system that allows for vital communication between parent and yourself to occur easily and frequently.

✧ Have the parents of the food-allergic child provide any and all food, or have only one person handing out the food in consultation with the food-allergic child's parents.

✧ Do not give food to a food-allergic child if there is any doubt regarding the safety of ingredients.

✧ Have an "offending ingredient free" lunch or food table, especially in environments with larger numbers of children.

✧ Substitute safe ingredients for offending ingredients in all craft projects or activities.

✧ Consider the safety of ingredients in food given to any class pets.

✧ Eliminate the offending food from the premises if at all possible. Consider the offending food as a loaded gun to the child at risk for experiencing a food-induced anaphylactic reaction.

✧ Take precautions even when the food-allergic child is not present to reduce the chance of cross-contamination.

✧ Have a "no food sharing " policy.

✧ Have the food-allergic child sit at the same place at mealtimes.

✧ Space toddlers in high chairs wide enough apart to eliminate the grabbing of one another's food.

✧ Have parents label bottles and food containers meant for the food-allergic child.

✧ Wipe hands and faces of other children before resuming play.

✧ Do not allow children to roam around with food. Eat in one area only.

✧ Include the food-allergic child as much as safely possible.

✧ Take special precautions at holiday or birthday celebrations.

✦ Do not allow a food-allergic child to eat what the parents of other children have brought in, unless the parents have spoken to a parent of the food-allergic child personally. Cross-contamination, misunderstandings, and hidden ingredients are common.

✦ Ask parents of the food-allergic child to chaperone all field trips, or, if this is not possible, assign one staff person to be solely responsible for recognizing and treating any potential allergic reactions. Research emergency medical care availability at the proposed site. Have a contingency plan. Bring extra epinephrine to allow additional time to reach a hospital emergency room.

RECOGNIZING AND TREATING AN ALLERGIC REACTION

As you know, food avoidance is the only sure way to prevent an allergic reaction. Being prepared to recognize and treat an allergic reaction is just as important.

Keep in mind that the time between exposure to an offending ingredient and the onset of symptoms can vary from two minutes to two hours, perhaps even longer. Even if a child has not been exposed while in your care, there is always a risk that a reaction could occur from an exposure earlier in the day. Also keep in mind that the types of symptoms, the severity of the symptoms, and the progression of the symptoms from a true allergic reaction can vary for each person. Even if in past exposures a child only vomited, there is no guarantee that the next exposure will not become a full-blown anaphylactic reaction. This is why caregivers must always be prepared to recognize and treat a reaction even if logic would dictate that a reaction would not occur. This is also why every reaction must be taken seriously, assessed carefully, and treated quickly.

BE PREPARED

Being prepared for an allergic reaction is vital. There are several things you can do to prepare yourself for this kind of emergency.

✧ Become acquainted with the child's history of reactions.

✧ Discuss and document the detailed emergency procedures for each child.

✧ Create a backup emergency plan.

✧ Have at least one EpiPen that stays on the premises in a safe but unlocked location, preferably in the same room as the child, and an additional EpiPen located in a central location.

✧ Post emergency procedures in a convenient and highly visible place.

✧ Educate all other people or staff about emergency procedures.

✧ Have a practice "reaction drill" periodically to refresh your memory of the proper procedures.

✧ Check expiration dates of the EpiPen and other medications periodically.

✧ Inform local rescue squads of the child's allergy and emergency treatment requirements. Inquire whether the rescue squad carries epinephrine.

✧ Periodically monitor and evaluate current methods of food avoidance, and improve and update as necessary.

✧ Periodically monitor and evaluate current emergency procedures, and improve and update as necessary.

Recognizing and treating an allergic reaction quickly and properly is vital. Check with the child's parents and/or doctor as to individual assessment guidelines. It is generally accepted that if *any one* of the following symptoms is experienced, the emergency plan should be put into action:

Feeling of anxiety or dread

Redness of skin and/or hives

Warmth and swelling of skin

Itching and/or swelling of lips, throat, and tongue

Itchy eyes, sneezing, coughing, hoarseness

Wheezing

Chest and throat tightness

Nausea, vomiting, abdominal cramps, diarrhea

Shortness of breath

Increased heart rate

Loss of consciousness due to rapid and severe drop in blood pressure

Alert others that the child is possibly experiencing an allergic reaction. Check to see if the child has had any new or suspicious foods, or, if the child is old enough, ask if any food ingested bothered him or her. If any new symptoms develop or if the reaction is clearly progressing, administer the EpiPen injection to the outer thigh area as soon as possible. Survival rates are directly linked to a prompt recognition of a reaction and the administration of the EpiPen before or at the *first* sign of any respiratory distress. Many physicians prescribe the use of an oral antihistamine such as Benadryl. The specific guidelines for administering a liquid antihistamine should be discussed with the child's physician.

Proceed by calling 911 if applicable, or immediately transport the child to the nearest hospital emergency room for further treatment. If transportation takes longer than the fifteen to twenty minutes of EpiPen efficacy or if the child's condition is clearly worsening, repeat the EpiPen as necessary. If it turns out that administering the EpiPen had not been necessary, no ill effects will be experienced to the child except the pain of the needle. The child and the parents of the child will most likely be thankful that you cared enough to take action. If it turns out that a child did need the EpiPen administered and you did not inject it, serious harm could have come to the child.

BEING EMOTIONALLY PREPARED

When caring for a child at risk for experiencing a food-induced anaphylactic reaction, it is hard to know what to expect. Knowledge usually comes in bits and pieces of alarming information gleaned from the experiences of others. Although living with unknowns can be very stressful, the experience may at least be made more predictable by mapping out the territory. Becoming aware of what you may experience may make the overwhelming task of caring for a food-allergic child seem more manageable.

When the aunt of a food-allergic child was asked about the issues that were relevant to her care for her five-year-old nephew, she immediately thought of the troubling dreams she experienced. She would sometimes awaken panic-stricken after dreaming that she had somehow forgotten her nephew's allergy, had given him an obviously offensive food, and was then literally paralyzed to take any emergency action as she watched her nephew's body swell. The feelings of fear, failure in her responsibility, concern for her nephew, and guilt were vivid to her.

Fear

Caring for a food-allergic child often produces deep emotions, including fear. It is normal to fear many things, including:

- ✧ The greatest of all fears, the death of a child who is in your care
- ✧ Forgetting to check ingredients or making a mistake that will cause the child to experience a severe allergic reaction

- Incorrectly assessing symptoms, resulting in an incorrect response
- Having to administer an injection and obtain further life-saving treatment for the child
- Having to contact the child's parents and inform them of a reaction
- Talking to the parents and child after an accidental reaction has occurred
- Being legally liable for an accidental ingestion

Responsibility

Parents and caregivers of food-allergic children bear an unusually high sense of responsibility. The stakes could not be higher than a child's life. It is a heavy burden to be responsible for:

✧ Preventing a reaction—management of food avoidance

✧ Recognizing a reaction

✧ Treating a reaction

Guilt

Guilt is an emotion that may be felt in many situations, including:

✧ When a child has been exposed to an offending ingredient while in your care, even if it was unavoidable, as when a product has been labeled incorrectly or cross-contamination has occurred

✧ Incorrectly assessing or recognizing a possible allergic reaction

✧ Waiting too long to begin treating a reaction

YOUR LEGAL LIABILITY

Potential legal liability is a common concern of caregivers. True, some caregivers never even consider their legal liability if the child has a reaction and they need to administer the EpiPen injection. However, other caregivers report potential liability as the leading reason why they would rather not care for a food-allergic child.

It is easy to understand why liability would be a troubling issue, especially if a business establishment is involved, such as a day care center, or if the adult caregiver does not know the food-allergic child's parents very well. But the reality of the situation is that there is every reason to provide safe care for the food-allergic child, and the reasons not to provide care may be based on fear or ignorance of food allergies.

Many professional child care providers or laypeople report never questioning *whether* they should provide care to a food-allergic child but *how* to do it safely. They believe every child has the inherent right to be cared for and every child brings into child care some issue that needs to be addressed. Food allergies happen to be the issue for some children. Some caregivers view the situation as a learning experience and enthusiastically become educated about food allergies and begin investigating how best to keep the child safe.

As mentioned in chapter 4, food-allergic children have legal rights entitling them to receive safe care, and refusing that child care may be legally unsound. All children have the right to care and protection. Although a "hidden" condition, food allergies are considered by some to be a disability in the eyes of the law. Section 504 of the Rehabilitation Act of 1973 defines a disability as a physical impairment that severely limits one or more major life activities such as breathing, eating, and going to school. Although the laws are sometimes conflicting, they can provide you with legal guidelines for caring for a child with food allergies. Children with disabilities are granted additional protection and rights under the Individuals with Disabilities Education Act and the Americans with Disabilities Act of 1990. These laws protect children's right to receive safe care in the "least restrictive" environment. The goal of this provision is the creation of child-driven programs and materials to be adapted to the child's needs in an effort to eliminate any segregation or deny the child full participation.

In the past, some caregivers have asked parents to sign a waiver of liability to protect themselves from any legal consequences for negligence or failure to provide emergency treatment. This effort to protect yourself is not foolproof, as courts may invalidate various waivers. For those caregivers still concerned about liability, the best protection is working with parents to create a formal written plan to minimize risks and to consult your own common sense. "There is serious risk to be managed, and the greatest exposure to risk comes when caregivers fail to do what is appropriate to protect a child," says Ellie Goldberg, M.Ed., educational rights specialist.

When arranging alternate care for their food-allergic child, the last thing on parents' minds is liability. They are looking for a willing and cooperative person who will see that their child is treated like every other child in almost every way, and take the necessary steps to ensure the child's safety, just as you would for a child without food allergies. Parents want to know that you will learn how to practice food avoidance, recognize if a reaction is occurring, and respond by providing emergency treatment if necessary. When you care for children, any one of them could experience an unexpected emergency, and caregivers would be responsible for responding. The difference is that with a food-allergic child you can prepare yourself for a possible anaphylactic reaction.

STANDING IN THE PARENTS' SHOES

Understanding the parents of a food-allergic child can be puzzling for some caregivers. Once a caregiver becomes fully educated about severe food allergies, it is suddenly evident where the parents' concern is coming from. Parents are sometimes perceived to be overprotective or "crazy." This protectiveness is understandable when you consider that their child's life is at stake.

Parents must do whatever they feel is necessary to help ensure their child's safety. Take this into consideration when dealing with parents of food-allergic children. Become a partner with the concerned parent—join in doing what the parent asks of you and come up with additional ways to minimize risks. If you react in a way that is unconcerned or uncooperative, the parent is likely to behave in a way that seems more unreasonable. When you react and follow through in a way that shows the parent that you understand what the parent has said about anaphylaxis, the parent will naturally de-escalate. Taking food allergies seriously and doing everything you can to keep the child safe will benefit everyone involved.

Occasionally after learning about serious food allergies, you may encounter a parent that you perceive to be underreacting. He or she may not carry an EpiPen, despite previous serious allergic reactions. The parent may not possess a full and accurate understanding of food allergies, or may not know how to communicate the child's needs.

A parent should not leave a food-allergic child without available treatment. Simply avoiding the offending foods has proven to be unreliable and has led to tragic results. Every reaction is different, and the fact that the child "only" developed hives or vomited during past allergic reactions does *not* mean that the next reaction, or the next, could not progress to a full-blown anaphylactic reaction. In this case you may want to recommend that the child see an allergist to determine whether previous reactions were due to a true food allergy, which involves the immune system. This can usually be determined through skin and blood tests, in addition to a complete medical evaluation. If a true food allergy exists, it is in the child's, as well as your, best interest to have an EpiPen on site.

Supporting Normal Developmental Needs

As discussed in chapter 4, parents may adapt the role they play in the management of their child's food allergy to the changing needs of their growing child. In providing care for the food-allergic child, it is important to understand what the parents' goals may be during the different stages of growth in order to support this necessary development.

Birth to Age Five

The very young food-allergic child requires parents and caregivers to take full control of management of food avoidance and recognition and treatment of reactions. The very small child cannot verbalize or fully comprehend his or her own needs. Small children will be dependent on others. During this stage, you and the parent cannot be too protective. Instead, provide "necessary protection" for the child. Support the parents in their quest to create the safest possible environment for their young food-allergic child. Accomplishing this may require approaches that are outside the normal paradigms of what other child care providers are doing. Support the parents in any way they wish to accomplish this. The parent may wish to remain present during a preschool class.

As they near age five, children need to begin to take age-appropriate control of their own allergies. Even very young children should have an awareness of their food allergies and begin to use the method of checking with adults before eating anything. This is the very foundation of the child's developing self-esteem.

Ages Five to Eleven

School-aged children are confronted with new and widening opportunities as their world begins to blossom. School cafeterias, slumber party invitations, field trips, and bus rides enter every child's world. While exciting, these new situations can be frightening for parents of a food-allergic child.

For the child's well-being and to respect the normal developmental process, five- to eleven-year-olds should be encouraged to take more responsibility for their own care. This will include communicating needs to others, reading food labels, and eventually being responsible for carrying the EpiPen and learning how to self-administer the injection, if absolutely necessary.

A conflict can arise in this stage of life when parents attempt to manage the child's allergies in the same ways they did when the child was three years old. Your job should be to support parents as they adopt new methods for creating the safest possible environment. This involves the beginning of a letting-go process that, for parents of children with life-threatening food allergies, can be extremely difficult.

During this stage, teasing and bullying of the food-allergic child by other children may become a problem. Children who have always accepted and managed their allergy remarkably well might respond by becoming angry about having to cope with their food allergy. This is normal and should be listened to and supported. You can help by encouraging a supportive environment and refusing to tolerate any teasing or bullying.

The Big Picture

There are many other things caregivers can do to support the food-allergic child's necessary development and growing self-esteem. During each stage it is your job in caring for the child to encourage and protect the growing self-esteem of the child. Food allergies can affect the normal developmental process of becoming an independent person, as well as jeopardizing a child's fragile self-esteem.

It is important for kids with food allergies to know and believe that having a food allergy is just one part of who they are. Encourage others to come to understand this by using the food allergies as a learning experience and do not dwell on them or draw attention to them unnecessarily. Include the food-allergic child as much as possible. Make substitutions or alter plans to avoid excluding the child from activities, outings, celebrations, or even daily meals.

I know it is difficult for caregivers to comprehend all the pertinent information about food allergies at one sitting. Parents certainly do not set out to scare you; however, you need to know everything in order to make good decisions regarding the care you provide. Take into consideration that you will not be dealing with everything contained in this chapter at one time. Realize your importance in your role, and take each challenge one at a time.

Providing safety to children with food allergies is manageable. You will quickly become a label reader and become more confident of your care every day. Each caregiver that I have ever had take care of my son has consistently remarked that providing a safe environment and managing the emotions associated with this responsibility become so much easier over time. In time, the methods you use to provide safety will become second nature, forging a powerful connection between you and the child.

RESOURCE GUIDE

———— ∼ ————

For more information on food allergies, contact:

The Food Allergy Network
10400 Eaton Place, Suite 107
Fairfax, VA 22030-2208
Phone (800) 929-4040 or (703) 691-3179
Fax (703) 691-2713
Visit their Web site *http://www.foodallergy.org*

A national nonprofit organization established to increase public awareness about food allergy and anaphylaxis. Provides education, emotional support, and coping strategies for individuals with food allergies. Send self-addressed stamped envelope for free sample quarterly newsletter.

Healthy Kids: The Key to Basics
Educational Planning for Students with Chronic Health Conditions
Ellie Goldberg, M.Ed., Educational Rights Specialist
79 Elmore Street
Newton, MA 02459-1137
Phone (617) 965-9637

Fax (617) 965-5407

e-mail erg_hk@juno.com

An information and consulting service created to improve understanding of the needs of children with chronic health concerns
and to share information about exemplary resources and programs. For more information on resources available, please send
$1 and a self-addressed stamped business envelope.

National Institutes of Health

Bethesda, MD 20892

Phone (301) 496-5343

Request NIH Publication No. 91-2650, *Managing Allergies and
Asthma at School: Tips for School Teachers and Staff,* a booklet that
describes how to recognize children who have allergies or
asthma, how to help them manage their condition at school while
avoiding making them feel different from other students, and how
to create a cooperative plan of care that establishes communication between home, school, and physician.

Asthma and Allergy Foundation of America

1125 West 15th Street, NW, Suite 502

Washington, DC 20005

Phone (800) 7-ASTHMA

National nonprofit organization dedicated to helping people with
asthma and allergic diseases. AAFA offers many services, including pamphlets, books, and videos. Local chapters provide support
groups.

American Lung Association

1740 Broadway

New York, NY 10019

Phone (800) LUNG-USA

Asthma is the leading serious chronic illness of all children in the United States; ALA's long-term goal is to implement its school-based asthma program, Open Airways for Schools, in every elementary school in the country. The ALA provides educational materials for individuals as well as teachers. Many chapters have asthma support groups or seminars.

National Information Center for Children and
  Youth with Handicaps
P.O. Box 1492
Washington, DC 20013
Phone (800) 695-0285

Free information to parents, educators, and child advocates.

For a list of allergists in your area, contact:

The American Academy of Allergy, Asthma, and Immunology
Phone (800) 822-ASMA
    or
The American College of Allergy, Asthma, and Immunology
Phone (800) 842-7777

Emergency medical identification organizations:

American Medical Identifications
(713) 695-0284 or (800) 363-5985

MedicAlert Foundation
(800) 825-3785

Medi-Guard I.D.
(800) 599-9757

Sta®Stat
(800) 943-9119

REFERENCES

———— ∾ ————

American Academy of Pediatrics. 1995. "Guidelines for Urgent Care in School." In A. Muñoz-Furlong, ed., *The School Food Allergy Program*. Fairfax, Va.: Food Allergy Network.

Bock, S. A. 1992. "The Incidence of Severe Adverse Reactions to Food in Colorado." *Journal of Allergy Clinical Immunology* 40: 683–85.

Bock, S. A., and F. M. Atkins. 1989. "The Natural History of Peanut Allergy." *Journal of Allergy and Clinical Immunology* 83: 900–904.

Bowen, M. 1978. *Family Therapy in Clinical Practice.* New York: Jason Aronson.

Brostoff, J. 1989. "Anaphylactic Reaction to Injected Hazelnut." *The Lancet* 8660: 459.

Canadian Society of Allergy and Clinical Immunology, Ontario Allergy Society, Allergy and Asthma Information Association. 1995. [Position paper] "Anaphylaxis in Schools and Other Child Care Settings."

Chase, M. 1995. "Peanut Allergies Have Put Sufferers on Alert." *Wall Street Journal,* Aug. 14.

Crain, W. 1992. *Theories of Development: Concepts and Applications.* 3d ed. Englewood Cliffs, N.J.: Prentice Hall.

Erikson, E. H. 1963. *Childhood and Society.* 2d ed. New York: W. W. Norton.

———. 1982. *The Life Cycle Completed.* New York: W. W. Norton.

Flatter, C. 1995. "Two To Five." In K. Ross, ed., "The Mother's Role." *Sesame Street Parents.* (May): 57–58.

Galt, V. 1995. "Severe Food Allergies Sticky Topic for Schools." *Boston Globe and Mail,* Sept. 23, pp. A1, A4.

Galyassy, M. 1995. "Harassment Stinks." *Food Allergy News* (4), (3), 1 & 3.

Goldberg, E. 1993. "The Americans with Disabilities Act: How Does It Affect You?" *Asthma and Allergy Foundation of America.* (Sept./Oct.): 6–7.

———. 1994. "School Liability Waivers." *Healthy Kids: The Key to Basics.* Newton, Mass.

Herzog, J. M., M.D., "Birth to Two." In K. Ross, ed., "The Mother's Role." *Sesame Street Parents.* (May): 57–58.

Hide, D.W., MB, FRCP, DCH. 1993. "Food-Induced Anaphylaxis—Death Can and Must Be Avoided" (letter to the editor). *British Journal of Clinical Practice* 47 (1): 6–7.

Hutchinson, B. 1995. "Kin: Eatery's Secret Recipe Killed Mom." *Boston Herald,* Aug. 7, pp. 1, 12.

Kantor, D., and W. Lehr. 1975. *Inside the Family.* San Francisco: Jossey-Bass.

Klein, N., M.D., and M. Lashley, M.D. 1990. "Case Report: Exercise-Induced Anaphylaxis in a 4-Year-Old Boy." *Annals of Allergy* 64: 381–82.

Levert, S. 1993. *Teens Face to Face with Chronic Illness.* New York: Messner.

Marinkovitch, V., M.D. 1992. Letter to the editor. *New England Journal of Medicine* 327 (25), pp. 1814–15.

Martindale, M. 1989. "A Joyful Outing Ends in Death for Girl on Class Trip." *Detroit News,* June 6.

Matloff, S., M.D. (Vol. 4, No. 1). Adverse Reactions to Food. *Asthma and Allergy Foundation Bulletin.*

Mendelson, L., M.D., J. P. Rosen, M.D., and H. A. Sampson, M.D. 1992. "Fatal and Near-Fatal Anaphylactic Reactions to Food in

Children and Adolescents." *New England Journal of Medicine* 327 (6), 380–84.

Muñoz-Furlong, A. 1995–96. "We're All in This Together." *Food Allergy News* (Dec.–Jan.): 2.

———. 1998. *Key Facts about the Food Allergy Network.* Fairfax, Va: The Food Allergy Network.

——— ed. 1995. *The School Food Allergy Program.* Fairfax, Va: The Food Allergy Network.

Rolland, J. S., M.D. 1994. *Families, Illness, and Disability: An Integrative Treatment Model.* New York: Basic Books.

Sampson, H., M.D., Scott Sicherer, M.D., Wesley Burks, M.D., and Ann Muñoz-Furlong. 1999. "Prevalence of Peanut and Tree Nut Allergy in the United States." *Journal of the American Academy of Allergy, Asthma, and Immunology* (April).

"Tony School KOs 5-Year-Old for Nutty Reason." 1995. *The Boston Herald,* April 15.

Segal, Michael, M.D. 1992. Letter to the editor. *New England Journal of Medicine* 327 (25): 1814–15.

Somerville, S. 1995. "Food Allergy Awareness: Decreasing the Danger Dining Out." *Restaurants USA* (Nov.), 35–38.

Taylor, S., Ph.D. 1995. "Choose Your Ice Cream Flavor Wisely." *Food Allergy News* (Feb.–Mar.): 7.

Understanding Food Allergy. 1993. (Brochure) American Academy of Allergy and Immunology.

White, M. 1989. *Selected Papers.* Adelaide, Australia: Dulwich Centre Publications.

Wowk, M. 1994. "Garbanzo Beans Kill Troy Girl." *Detroit News,* Feb. 10, p. 1B.

Yunginger, J. W., M.D. 1992. "Lethal Food Allergy in Children" (letter to the editor). *New England Journal of Medicine* 327 (6), 421–22.

INDEX

———— ⁓ ————

ABOUT THE AUTHOR

Lisa Cipriano Collins is the founder and president of Food Allergy Matters, specializing in consultation to families and various systems to provide information and support regarding the practical and emotional aspects of managing a child's food allergy. She was appointed to, and served as a volunteer on, the Member Advisory Council and Speaker's Bureau of the Food Allergy Network, a national nonprofit organization based in Fairfax, Virginia, the most prominent advocate for families affected by food allergies. She is a marriage and family therapist and has a private practice in Burlington, Massachusetts, where she resides with her husband and three children.

The author offers personal and professional consultations and group workshops regarding the management of food allergies in children. You may contact her at:

Lisa Cipriano Collins, M.A., M.F.T.

127 Cambridge St.

Burlington, MA 01803

Phone (781) 270-4945

Fax (781) 270-7856

e-mail cipcoll@rcn.com